Working With Chimps

THE DEVOLUTION OF AMERICAN HEALTHCARE

———

PJ NATHAN

Copyright © 2017 PJ Nathan
All rights reserved.

ISBN: 1542682185
ISBN 13: 9781542682183
Library of Congress Control Number: 2017900984
CreateSpace Independent Publishing Platform
North Charleston, South Carolina

Working With Chimps

*Vicki ~
Say hello to my
little book!
Love you Sister ~
Patty
April 2017*

Disclaimer

—

THE AUTHOR AND PUBLISHER HAVE made every effort to ensure that the information in this book is correct, and do not assume and hereby disclaim any liability to any party for any loss, damage, or disruption caused by errors or omissions, whether such errors or omissions result from inattention, accident, or any other cause.

Furthermore, the author and publisher would like to expressly convey to you, the reader, that were the author and publisher to accidently defame, purge, humiliate and/or hurt someone's person or feelings as a result of them reading, and/or acting upon any or all of the information, and/or advice found in this work, is entirely inadvertent.

Most importantly, it is not our intention to insult or offend the Chimpanzee.

Dedication

For every victim and survivor; you are never truly alone.

Table of Contents

Preface xi

Chapter 1   The Promise 1
Chapter 2   Who's Minding the Store? 10
Chapter 3   King Kong 17
Chapter 4   Drinking the Kool-Aid 23
Chapter 5   Community Life 38
Chapter 6   New Chimp 46
Chapter 7   Bad Chimp 70
Chapter 8   Sad Chimp 80
Chapter 9   Glad Chimp 107
Chapter 10 America's Present and Future
             State of Health 112

Acknowledgements 123
About the Author 125
Endnotes 127

Preface

"Most primates, including humans, spend their lives in large social groups or communities. [These] communities usually avoid each other and are aggressive towards outsiders."[1]

This statement applies to nearly every hospital in which I have worked. It has been said that "nurses eat their young." However, it seems lately that nurses, in general, are feasting upon older, more experienced colleagues rather than the young ones. Numerous facilities have taken the eating of the young to an entirely new level and, in many workplaces, this practice has evolved into outright denigration and bullying by colleagues, managers, and administrators.

The healthcare community is developing a new breed of autocratic leaders who model Standards of *Mis*behavior, yet command their subordinates to do as they say, not as they do. Add this phenomenon to the gradual decline of healthcare delivery systems overall, and the result is the loss of compassion as healthcare progressively trades beneficence for business.

This is a work based on truth. It is a collection of decades of nursing experience, illustrating the decline of American healthcare. I haven't named or shamed institutions or individuals directly in order to protect the guilty because, "Every man is guilty of all the good he did not do" (Voltaire). It is a sad commentary that, in today's society, we have to protect the guilty at the expense of the innocent.

PJ Nathan
March 2013

The Promise

---

*"People of integrity do what's right,
whether anybody is watching or not."*

~ JOEL OSTEEN

EVERY PHYSICIAN, PHYSICIAN ASSISTANT, NURSE practitioner, and registered and practical nurse recites their respective oath at the closing of their graduation ceremony. The oath is a pledge that describes the practitioner's commitment to future professional behavior. These promises form the foundation of business administrators and healthcare providers' tenets, and are principles to keep in mind as you read through this text. Here are the respective promises in full:

The Promise

Hippocratic Oath: Modern Version

Today's contemporary Hippocratic Oath [originally penned in the late 5th century BC], written in 1964 by Louis Lasagna, Academic Dean of the School of Medicine at Tufts University, is currently used in many medical schools.

> I swear to fulfill, to the best of my ability and judgment, this covenant:
> I will respect the hard-won scientific gains of those physicians in whose steps I walk, and gladly share such knowledge as is mine with those who are to follow.
> I will apply, for the benefit of the sick, all measures [that] are required, avoiding those twin traps of overtreatment and therapeutic nihilism.
> I will remember that there is an art to medicine as well as science, and that warmth, sympathy, and understanding may outweigh the surgeon's knife or the chemist's drug.
> I will not be ashamed to say "I know not," nor will I fail to call in my colleagues when the skills of another are needed for a patient's recovery.
> I will respect the privacy of my patients, for their problems are not disclosed to me that

the world may know. Most especially, I must
tread with care in matters of life and death.
If it is given me to save a life, all thanks. But
it may also be within my power to take a life;
this awesome responsibility must be faced
with great humbleness and awareness of my
own frailty. Above all, I must not play at God.
I will remember that I do not treat a fever
chart, a cancerous growth, but a sick human being, whose illness may affect the
person's family and economic stability. My
responsibility includes these related problems, if I am to care adequately for the sick.
I will prevent disease whenever I can,
for prevention is preferable to cure.
I will remember that I remain a member of society, with special obligations to
all my fellow human beings, those sound
of mind and body as well as the infirm.
If I do not violate this oath, may I enjoy
life and art, respected while I live and remembered with affection thereafter.
May I always act to preserve the finest traditions of my calling and may I long experience
the joy of healing those who seek my help.[2]

The Promise

Physician Assistant Professional Oath

I pledge to perform the following duties with honesty and dedication:
I will hold as my primary responsibility the health, safety, welfare and dignity of all human beings.
I will uphold the tenets of patient autonomy, beneficence, nonmaleficence and justice.
I will recognize and promote the value of diversity.
I will treat all persons who seek my care
I will hold in confidence the information shared in the course of practicing medicine.
I will assess my personal capabilities and limitations, striving always to improve my medical practice.
I will actively seek to expand my knowledge and skills, keeping abreast of advances in medicine.
I will work with other members of the health care team to provide compassionate and effective care of patients.
I will use my knowledge and experience to contribute to an improved community.

I will respect my professional relationship with the physician.
I will share and expand knowledge within the profession.
These duties are pledged with sincerity and upon my honor.[3]

Florence Nightingale Pledge
(Registered Nurse)

I solemnly pledge myself before God and in the presence of this assembly, to pass my life in purity and to practice my profession faithfully.
I will abstain from whatever is deleterious and mischievous, and will not take or knowingly administer any harmful drug.
I will do all in my power to maintain and elevate the standard of my profession, and will hold in confidence all personal matters committed to my keeping and all family affairs coming to my knowledge in the practice of my calling.
With loyalty will I endeavor to aid the physician in his work, and devote myself to the welfare of those committed to my care.[4]

Practical Nurse Pledge

> Before God and those assembled here, I solemnly pledge to adhere to the code of ethics of the nursing profession;
> To cooperate faithfully with the other members of the nursing team and to carry out faithfully and to the best of my ability the instructions of the physician or the nurse who may be assigned to supervise my work;
> I will not do anything evil or malicious and I will not knowingly give any harmful drug or assist in malpractice;
> I will not reveal any confidential information that may come to my knowledge in the course of my work;
> And I pledge myself to do all in my power to raise the standards and prestige of practical nursing.
> May my life be devoted to service and to the high ideals of the nursing profession.[5]

The Master of Business Administration (MBA) oath "is a voluntary [optional] student-led pledge that asks graduating MBAs to commit towards the creation of value "responsibly and ethically." As of January 2010, the initiative is driven by a coalition of MBA students, graduates, and advisors, including nearly 2,000 student and alumni signers from over 500 MBA programs around the world. By formalizing a written oath and creating forums for individuals to personally commit to an ethical standard, the initiative hopes to accomplish three goals:

1. To make a difference in the lives of individual students who take the oath
2. To challenge other classmates to work towards a higher professional standard, whether they sign the oath or not, and
3. To create a public conversation in the press about professionalizing and improving management"[6]

The MBA Oath

As a business leader I recognize my role in society.

- My purpose is to lead people and manage resources to create value that no single individual can create alone.
- My decisions affect the well-being of individuals inside and outside my enterprise today and tomorrow.

Therefore, I promise that:

- I will manage my enterprise with loyalty and care, and will not advance my personal interests at the expense of my enterprise or society.
- I will understand and uphold, in letter and spirit, the laws and contracts governing my conduct and that of my enterprise.
- I will refrain from corruption, unfair competition, or business practices harmful to society.
- I will protect the human rights and dignity of all people affected by my enterprise, and I will oppose discrimination and exploitation.
- I will protect the right of future generations to advance their standard of living and enjoy a healthy planet.
- I will report the performance and risks of my enterprise accurately and honestly.
- I will invest in developing myself and others, helping the management profession continue to advance and create sustainable and inclusive prosperity.

> In exercising my professional duties according to these principles, I recognize that my behavior must set an example of integrity, eliciting trust and esteem from

those I serve. I will remain accountable to my peers and to society for my actions and for upholding these standards.

This oath I make freely, and upon my honor.[7]

An extensive search reveals that there is currently no relevant healthcare professional Baccalaureate program (other than an undergraduate nursing degree) that requires a conscious guiding vow.

Who's Minding the Store?

"How do you suppose I got to be the general manager of this great store?"[8]

THE NATIONAL ASSOCIATION OF PUBLIC Hospitals (2009) describes the origins of today's hospitals in the following excerpt:

> In the early nineteenth century, and for more than a century to come, most Americans gave birth and endured illness and even surgery at home. They belonged to a largely rural society, and few among them would ever have occasion to visit a hospital. Hospitals in the United States emerged from institutions, notably almshouses, that provided care and custody

for the ailing poor. Rooted in this tradition of charity, the public hospital traces its ancestry to the development of cities and community efforts to shelter and care for the chronically ill, deprived, and disabled. A six-bed ward founded in 1736 in the New York City Almshouse became, over the course of a century and more, *Bellevue Hospital*. The predecessor of *Charity Hospital* in New Orleans opened its doors the same year. Today's *Regional Medical Center* in Memphis, the oldest hospital in Tennessee, was founded in 1829. Similar origins exist for other public hospitals — places where the "care of strangers" grew from modest origins into multifaceted municipal institutions.[9]

It is interesting to note that "early hospital administrators were called 'superintendents' and typically had little specific training for their jobs — many were nurses who had taken on administrative responsibilities."[10] Despite the first established hospital and nursing school administration health economics program (in 1900) at New York's Columbia Teachers College, physicians, laypersons, and Catholic sisters continued to oversee operations as superintendents (Stevens, 1999).

Over a century later, the practice of utilizing underprepared nurses as managers and supervisors, and unqualified administrators as hospital leaders, continues to be the standard. Incredibly, the United States Bureau of Labor Statistics supports this archaic stance with their statement that "work experience in a related occupation…is a commonly accepted substitute for more formal types of training or education."

Although many institutions currently require a Bachelor or Master's degree for certain managerial positions, additional formal *leadership* education is frequently substituted for an arbitrary number of "years of experience." Those years of experience refer to how much time a professional has spent doing a particular set of tasks, in a particular department, for no healthcare employer in particular. The job becomes so routine it brings to mind the adage, "even a monkey can do that job."

Leaders are not born, they are developed. And while leadership training does not guarantee successful management, it does provide the candidate an opportunity to understand the core principles of this essential healthcare function. Additionally, leadership training may help a person determine if they are cut out for this type of responsibility.

As hospitals evolved, "nurse 'superintendents' were replaced with physicians that, in turn, prompted hospitals to be routinely led by doctors. That has [since] changed."[11]

According to IZA Institute for the Study of Labor (2011) Senior Research Associate Amanda H. Goodall:

> In the United Kingdom (UK) and the United States (US), most hospital chief executive officers (CEOs) are non-physician managers rather than physicians. Of the 6,500 hospitals in the US, only 235 are led by physicians (Gunderman & Kanter, 2009). It has been suggested that placing physicians into leadership positions can result in improved hospital performance and patient care. Some outstanding American medical facilities — for example the Cleveland and Mayo Clinics — have explicitly introduced leadership training, and management and leadership education is being incorporated into medical degrees. Currently, however, there are no empirical studies that assess the physician-leadership hypothesis that hospitals perform better when they are led by doctors.[12]

However, as Carl Sagan reminds us, "The absence of evidence is not the evidence of absence."

Since its early beginnings, healthcare has evolved tremendously throughout the decades. Great strides have been made in research, technology, accessibility to medical services, and so on, resulting in many more lives being saved. Provider focus is trending toward a person's health rather than their hospitalization, which empowers the patient as they partner with their healthcare giver.

Conversely, the advent of today's "multifaceted institutions" has shaken the very core of medicine and nursing. Provider motivation, behavior, morals, and ethics are often compromised by cost-cutting, and other fiscal demands and incentives imposed upon them by those operating the business of healthcare. It is nearly impossible to maintain the original altruistic foundation of healthcare in today's revenue-conscious health delivery systems.

Healthcare is big corporate business with the profit margin, not patient care, being its main objective; it is "America's largest industry by far, employing a sixth of the country's workforce. And it is the average American family's largest single expense, whether paid out of their pockets or through taxes and insurance premiums" (Brill, 2015). The devolution of healthcare began around the end of the 20th century and has never looked back. These changes have been insidious; however, recent federal legislation and reimbursement requirements blatantly threaten to compromise the health and well-being of all Americans.

It might benefit the government and healthcare administrators to realize that, as Winston Churchill cautioned, "However beautiful the strategy, you should occasionally look at the results." I believe there can be a healthy balance between business and beneficence without compromising either corporate or medical ethics. Unfortunately, that happy medium has yet to manifest, as the scales of social justice continue to lean woefully toward a company's balance sheet.

Much like the un-trained nurse "superintendent" of centuries ago, the majority of today's hospital chief executive officers (CEOs) have a Bachelor's degree at best. According to Forbes et al., of the nearly 22 million CEOs, 47% have a Bachelor's degree, 25% a Master's and 2% have a Ph.D. Furthermore, 66% of CEOs are promoted internally.[13]

Many of these Baccalaureate CEOs have irrelevant undergraduate degrees in non-business and non-healthcare sciences. Imagine a situation in which you have a contracted college graduate, with no advanced degree, roaming the building. After a few years, the hospital loses its chief operating officer (COO). The contracted employee has been around for a few years, is familiar with the organization and has an education of sorts, so the hospital hires them and puts them in charge of operations. Then a few years later they need a CEO. The person with the Bachelor's degree who's worked in the hospital for several more years surely must be qualified by now to run the organization; after all, they've worn a few hats so they must know *something* about how to manage a hospital. A CEO is born; and again, we're back to monkeys.

King Kong

"Neither man nor beast, but something monstrous."[14]

THE HIERARCHY WITHIN A CHIMP community is determined by the position and influence the creature has on others within the group. Similarly, the hierarchy of a corporation is arranged according to an individual's job function and authority.

Typical American hospital administrators are those in the C-suite who are responsible for operating an entire organization, whereas managers are accountable for running a specific company department. At the top of a hospital's multi-level "chief" hierarchy is the CEO (chief executive officer or president) followed by other C-level administrators such as a CHRO (human resources), COO (operations), CFO (finance), CNO (nursing), and other C-acronyms.

Alongside the CEO, upper management is reserved for the appointed physician Medical Director, who is chosen from one of the medical services "chiefs" such as Chief of Surgery, Chief of Medicine, Chief of Emergency Services, and so on. Generally, one Medical Director oversees the other physician department directors, or chiefs.

Further discussion regarding the role of Medical Director, and their staff, is limited since the CEO has the final word in most all hospital practices (the exception being those facilities in which a community represented board of trustees or commissioners is the figurehead to whom the CEO theoretically answers). It is my observation that beginning around the end of the last century, the physician and their directors receive little acknowledgement, and input is typically ignored, unless it is an ingenious cost-saving revelation.

Next in the chain of command is middle management, who directly answers to those in the C-suite. These managers oversee their respective departments and are the first in the chain of a subordinate's command. Lower management, also known as house supervisors, follows department managers.

Visually, this can be seen as:

Generic Hospital Organizational Chart Example

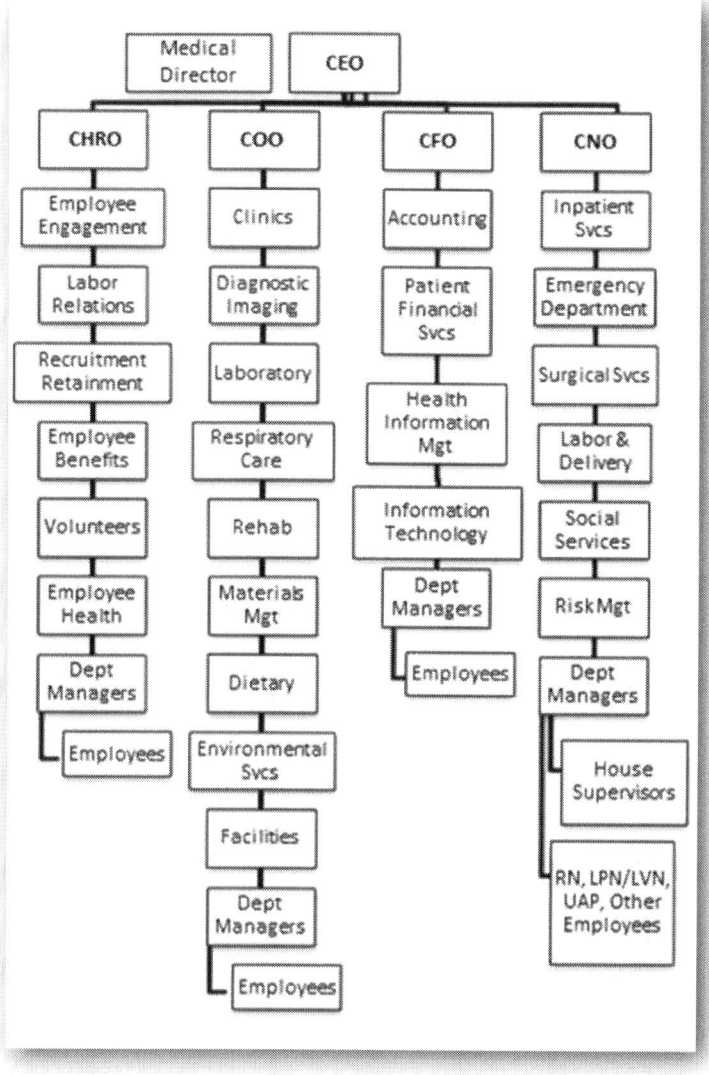

Lastly, there are the employees in each department who are theoretically further broken down into varying levels of experience and authority. However, no matter how artfully the corporation glamorizes the employee's role, the employee is the one who performs the actual labor for the organization and facilitates the institution's existence.

"The way administrators say it is (left), is not always the way it works (right)."[15]

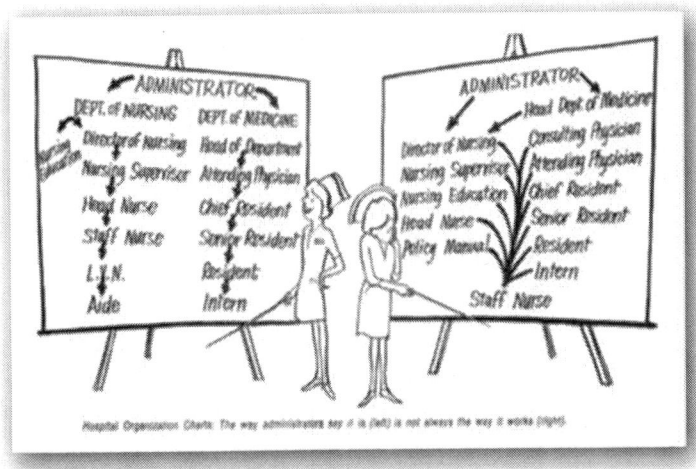

Chimps live in a male dominated hierarchy, whereas in a human corporate structure, males *and* females may govern. Regardless of gender, much like the dominant chimp hierarchy "where the alpha often charges and 'displays' by bristling his hair, dragging or shaking branches and banging or stomping on whatever he can find,"[16] healthcare administrators tend to ape the antagonistic behaviors of their primate counterparts — often in cinematic proportions.

Just as "these displays serve to make a male chimpanzee look large and powerful, often more so than he may actually be,"[17] so it is in healthcare administration. In their attempt to maintain control of their authoritative responsibilities, administrators often end up wreaking havoc in their wake.

Administrators oversee operations, make policies, and demand perpetuation of their many expectations. Department managers and supervisors achieve these executive directives by modeling their administrators' behaviors, and enforcing rules and hospital standards.

I've worked in many facilities where the culture of administrative impropriety gradually evolves into predictable staff conformity. I have also observed situations in which employee obedience is accomplished through mandates and the threat of severe reprimand, especially to those who practice within the moral code of their profession rather than compromise their integrity by kowtowing to the manipulative and calculating powers that be.

As in the chimpanzee world, corporate America has its alpha leaders and subordinates. Although the employee has little say in departmental and hospital processes, their input is often deceptively welcomed. Where did your idea go? Check your bosses' circular file. Yep, employees have little to no say — unless they drink the Kool-Aid.

Drinking the Kool-Aid

"For people will be lovers of self, lovers of money, proud, arrogant, abusive…unholy, heartless, unappeasable, slanderous, without self-control, brutal, not loving good, treacherous, reckless, swollen with conceit…AVOID SUCH PEOPLE."

~ II TIMOTHY 3:2-5 [ESV]

RECENT RESEARCH FINDINGS DEMONSTRATE THAT chimps share similar personality traits with their human cousins. The Public Library of Science (2014) explains that even though "primate personality psychology is a relatively new research area, initial studies reveal that chimps have two major similar human traits: the dominant Alpha and the more social Beta. These characteristics are broken down into smaller traits and paralleled with the five major human behaviors of openness, conscientiousness, extraversion, agreeableness, and neuroticism." This is where the chimp personality comparisons stop since humanesque personality *disorders* have yet to be studied.

As research studies continue, primate and human personality trait similarities may be modified however, the fact that we humans share about 98% of our DNA with chimps will not likely change; there will always be that 2% which distinguishes "us" from "them." And that may not always be a good thing.

Drinking the Kool-Aid is a disturbing psychological strategy of control and dominance that only a deviant human psyche is capable of creating and executing. It refers to the 1978 Guyana cult mass-suicide, the Jonestown Massacre, where 913 of the 1100 Jonestown residents drank potassium cyanide-laced Kool-Aid and died. Although "drinking the Kool-Aid is a figure of speech... [it] refers to a person or group holding an unquestioned belief, argument, or philosophy without critical examination."[18]

This practice is prevalent in a healthcare setting in which there is typical autocratic control. The morally disengaged executive's goal is to create a cult-like community of subordinates who are devoted to them. These are the leaders who convince themselves that ethics, and their professional oath, no longer applies to them as "they separate moral reactions from [their] inhumane conduct by disabling the mechanism of self-condemnation" (Fiske, 2004).

There are three types of unprincipled people in the business of healthcare. Those who:

1. Make the Kool-Aid.
2. Serve the Kool-Aid.
3. Drink the Kool-Aid.

Those who make the Kool-Aid live in the C-suite. They distribute it to middle and lower management who, in turn, serve it to the employee. Employees who decline the Kool-Aid are eventually filtered out of the system by either termination or resignation. Those who drink the Kool-Aid are deceptively reassured of long-term employment that, like low doses of ingestible cyanide, can be a very slow death.

The Kool-Aid makers demand blind obedience to their delusion of power and control. One of the C-suites' goals is that subordinates unconditionally accept their policies and standards, and that these edicts be disseminated to all employees. Intuitively, it may be supposed that the main motivation for these administrators is ego, power over and control of others, and of course money. Research verifies that these impressions are accurate.

Oliver James, a British clinical and occupational psychologist, author, and journalist identified three types of distinct dysfunctional personalities among white-collar workers: Narcissism, Machiavellianism, and Psychopathy.

Wikipedia provides a simple definition of these three dysfunctional personalities:

- Narcissism is characterized by grandiosity, pride, egotism, and a lack of empathy.
- Machiavellianism is characterized by manipulation and exploitation of others, a cynical disregard for morality, and a focus on self-interest and deception.
- Psychopathy is characterized by enduring antisocial behavior, impulsivity, selfishness, callousness, and remorselessness.[19]

Oliver James concluded that a fourth dysfunctional personality type, the "triadic person," is a combination of all three. He describes these "colleagues [as those] who have no compunction about trampling over others, or like nothing more than to plot and scheme, or drone on endlessly about themselves."[20] Furthermore, "those who display the most selfishness and deviousness rise to the top and narcissistic and Machiavellian tendencies thrive in the workplace. Such staff...have a dangerous, yet effective mix of self-centeredness, deviousness, self-regard and lack of empathy, which can propel them to the top of organisatians. The system you are in is liable to reward ruthless, selfish manipulation."[21]

To further simplify these traits, the triadic person is also termed the Dark Triad. As changingminds.org explains:

> The Dark Triad is a group of three personality traits, each of which may be considered not only anti-social but socially dangerous, as the person affected not only ignores the feelings of others but will use and abuse people for their own ends. In their need for control and identity, they ignore social values.

The three characteristics of the Dark Triad are:

- Narcissism: Seeks praise.
- Machiavellianism: The end justifies the means.
- Psychopathy: Seeks control.[22]

Not all leaders make Kool-Aid; there are many facilities whose bosses are principled, have integrity, and strive to guide the employee to his or her full potential. These are the people who model moral and ethical behaviors that inspire employees — which is what a leader should do. These leaders not only talk the talk; they walk the walk. It has been said that you cannot lead where you haven't been, and I have worked with many great leaders who have been there, done that and, with ongoing leadership training, have successfully transitioned through the ranks.

It's the Machiavellians, who demand a "do as I say, not as I do" edict, that give the C-suite a dark name. In so doing, they sublimate the needs of others with their own desires. The wise C-Mach (as in Machiavellian) knows better than to drink their own Kool-Aid, for as deep as their psychopathy runs, their narcissistic compulsion to succeed runs deeper.

In order to serve the Kool-Aid, middle and lower management must first buy into the scheme. Like those in the C-suite, these department managers and supervisors also fall into the Dark Triad category. I call these people mini-Machs; they haven't made it to the C-level but, like their administrators, their focus is on their own goals and agendas.

These middle and lower manager mini-Machs have their own narcissistic sense of entitlement, superiority, and dominance. Like their C-superiors, they are extremely motivated to elevate themselves, and often see the Kool-Aid as an opportunity for advancement, even though they have little to no inherent leadership abilities.

Leadership and workplace communication expert, speaker, author, and consultant Merge Gupta-Sunderji confirms that much of a superior's qualifications are in anything but management:

> Most people get promoted to supervisor or manager because they have a track record of results. They were accomplished at getting things done, and the eventual reward for their good work was the title of "manager." [One] critical fact that many people simply don't realize [is] all the skills and behaviours that make you successful as an individual contributor are also the very skills that will cause you to fail as a leader. ...thousands of supervisors and managers set themselves up to fail as leaders because they don't know that the new occupation called "leader" requires different skills and behaviors than what created success for them in the past. First, understand that your job satisfaction [as a leader] becomes more vicarious and intangible. In the past, you could take a task from beginning to end and enjoy the gratification that came from a job well done. And you might have even been publicly or privately

recognized for your efforts. As a leader, satisfaction now comes from watching members of your team take projects from start to finish, and rather than receiving recognition, it's your job to give it. Your sense of accomplishment must now come from seeing others grow and develop...[23]

It is important to keep in mind that a leadership presence should not be confused with leadership. In general, mini-Machs are life-long followers, and a major factor in their ineffective management may be attributed to their "inability to fulfill their job responsibilities" (Field, 1996). If they were effective leaders they would never drink, much less serve, the Kool-Aid.

Some Kool-Aid drinkers are wannabe mini-Machs whom I consider minions, while others are just natural born followers who will jump on any hierarchical bandwagon. This employee mix of minions and followers are both predisposed to similar mini-Mach thoughts and behaviors and, although they have no real power, minions and followers are eager to do their bosses' bidding. Minions, in their grandiose narcissistic state, may sincerely believe this is a stepping-stone toward the ladder of advancement. Followers may also believe they will be recognized and rewarded; however, I suspect their main objective is simply to keep their job. From here forward, both minions and followers will be collectively known as minions.

Now, there are also people who refuse to drink the Kool-Aid. Some are forced to voluntarily terminate their own employment through constructive discharge, but many continue working despite the oppression. Non-Kool-Aid drinkers are the principled employees who sincerely believe they can survive a grim work environment. I think of them as Nightingales. They assume they can make a difference and believe that the corporate situation will improve.

While Nightingales perform selfless duties that are guided by their training, competency, and professional code of ethics (not to mention the oath they took), mini-Machs and minions do everything in their power to undermine, sabotage, and denigrate the Nightingales. Kool-Aid drinkers are self-centric, and their latent insecurities make them uncomfortable with anyone who poses a perceived threat to their professional status. They tend to create, then home in on a Nightingale's fears, and relentlessly perpetuate their victim's increasing insecurities.

It is not unusual for mini-Machs (bosses) and minions (peers) to collaborate and strategize. Together they methodically feed the Nightingale's anxiety through repeated humiliation, embarrassment, ostracism, and other forms of emotional deconstruction, often with the unspoken threat of losing their job. Cultural anthropologist Janice Harper, Ph.D. (2013) describes how a seemingly innocuous verbal or non-verbal action can escalate into outright workplace terrorism:

> The signs a mob [also known as a group of bullies] is forming include any action on the part of management to formally criticize, investigate, warn, suspend, terminate or report a worker for wrongdoing. It may take the form of a harsh evaluation, a verbal rebuke, or a formal charge of misconduct. Leadership [as well as peers] ...will not waste any time alerting the workforce that the worker they want out is a trouble maker, "with a long history of issues/complaints/what-have-yous" who will be better off in another job. When this happens, even workers with stellar reputations and work records quickly find their identities and work histories revised as management discretely shares their concerns about the worker to the worker's coworkers, suggesting that opportunities for advancement or improved working conditions may ensue once the "difficult employee" is gone.[24]

Mini-Machs and minions seem to enjoy a sadistic satisfaction in their systematic destruction of others by denying Nightingales their employee rights and professional opportunities. In some cases, a Nightingale's very freedom to earn a living may be destroyed because the conspiracy to ruin their reputation until they become unemployable is that powerful, especially in close-knit and rural communities. The result is often a fight-or-flight stress response in which the Nightingale either becomes defensive and assertive, or intimidated and afraid; neither of which bode well for the Nightingale's holistic health and well-being, nor the patients being served. Dr. Cynthia Howard explains, "…perspective and…problem solving [are] not accessible when you are in a chronic stress mode."[25]

The Mayo Clinic emphasizes, "stress symptoms may be affecting your health, even though you might not realize it. You may think illness is to blame for that nagging headache, your frequent insomnia or your decreased productivity at work. But stress may actually be the culprit." They further explain how "stress symptoms can affect your body, your thoughts and feelings, and your behavior. Stress that's left unchecked can contribute to health problems, such as high blood pressure, heart disease, obesity and diabetes," and describe the common effects of stress:

1. On Your Body
   * Headache
   * Muscle tension or pain
   * Chest pain
   * Fatigue
   * Change in sex drive
   * Stomach upset
   * Sleep problems
2. On Your Mood:
   * Anxiety
   * Restlessness
   * Lack of motivation or focus
   * Irritability or anger
   * Sadness or depression
3. On Your Behavior:
   * Overeating or undereating
   * Angry outbursts
   * Drug or alcohol abuse
   * Tobacco use
   * Social withdrawal[26]

If there are no scrupulous senior staff and management around to curb hostile behavior, then that which begins as an occasional unapologetic incivility (an eye-roll here, a rude comment there) can lead to a widespread culture of bullying and blame. Nightingales have little to no recourse even though the organization may have an employee "harassment" policy. Should a Nightingale choose to report a policy violation by following the hierarchal chain-of-command, they are most often viewed as the perpetrator because blame is almost always shifted to the bully's victim.

Bullies don't apologize; they rationalize, and deflect their guilt by demonizing their target. Therefore, the Nightingale is the one who is often deemed as antagonizing, aggressive, and the actual cause of the problem, much in the same manner as those judging a rape victim — the thought process being that somehow the victim incited the unwelcomed actions of another because of the victim's 'unseemly' behavior.

Although acts of lateral violence among coequal colleagues (i.e. manager-to-manager) do happen, there have been concerns voiced by, or on the behalf of, management that bosses can become targets of subordinate bullying or mobbing. Ascending vertical violence may occur; however, it must be remembered that the superior holds a position of power and has the authority to stop it. A boss can document employee behavior, performance, and so on (whether it's true or fabricated), initiate a progressive discipline process and, if all else fails, the manager often has the option to transfer, and even terminate, the 'offending' employee(s). Unlike bullied subordinates who have little to no recourse, bosses who claim they are being bullied by their underlings does not hold a lot of water.

Contrary to these commonly accepted negative work-place behaviors, RN's are expected to follow the American Nurses Association *Nurse's Code of Ethics* that guides their professional conscience in maintaining the integrity of their practice. Every state's *Nurse Practice Act* further delineates what are and are not acceptable practice standards, defines professional behavioral expectations, and outlines each state's Board of Nursing reporting requirements for those who have knowledge of violations.

Mini-Machs and minions who abuse their authority and terrorize colleagues qualify as moral deviants and are, in my experience, an abomination to their profession. Repeated targeting, harassment, and mistreatment of employees are not prohibited according to a state's Board of Nursing, or any state or federal law…yet.

The day is coming when workplace bullying will be professionally prohibited and criminally illegal. Since 2003 more than half of the fifty American states have introduced the Healthy Workplace Bill[27]; however, it remains stalled in the labyrinth that is our legislative process. Despite the lack of an anti-bullying statute, Colson Center President John Stonestreet emphasizes that, "The legal status of something does not change its moral status, nor does it change our responsibility to the truth."

If any one thing is to be learned from this chapter it is that bosses can be a pathetic people, and I sometimes wonder if corporations might be better served if chimps actually did take over.[28]

Community Life

---

*"All animals are competitive by nature and
cooperative only under specific circumstances."*

~ FRANS DE WAAL

WHILE MINI-MACHS AND MINIONS CONTINUE to create an extremely difficult, hostile, and tense work environment, a façade of cooperation and teamwork must be present in order to sustain the facility's existence. Teamwork is a guiding principle for survival and is similar to a chimp community where all members know each other and work together for the good of the group. Although coordination and collaboration are vital to a group's ability to function effectively, trust is the glue that secures a team's success and community confidence.

According to Goodall (1986), Chapman et al. (1993), and Boesch (1996):

Chimps live in a fusion-fission social group consisting of a large community that includes all individuals that regularly associate with one another and smaller temporary subgroups. These subgroups are unpredictable and can be highly fluid, changing members quickly or lasting a few days before rejoining the community.[29]

Much like our primate counterparts, the healthcare community is a fusion-fission subculture of our global society. Although we may come and go as we please, we remain creatures of habit who function best with a measure of routine, order, and stability in our professional lives.

When the fusion-fission component is inconsistent or unpredictable, groups tend to become unstable. Therefore, when someone upsets our professional banana cart, the ability to perform effectively and efficiently can be lost, and chaos may ensue. If the turmoil persists, this instability will most assuredly seep into our personal lives as well. Resolution should be the priority in order to prevent a catastrophic flood of professional, communal, and personal mayhem. Corrective measures are imperative for survival; if not implemented, then when one domino falls, the entire structure will eventually collapse.

A healthcare community's survival depends upon its leaders to maintain its existence. Unfortunately, there are many facilities whose organizational leaders "encourage and support practices that produce unprofessional, unproductive, or incompetent managers" (Gilley & Boughton, 1996). Once the seeds of managerial malpractice are planted, the roots of malfeasance begin to bloom and rapidly spread throughout the organization. A toxic work environment leads to detrimental and often devastating patient outcomes due to its negative effect on the employee's motivation and performance. Low employee morale creates a culture of strife, discord, and division which leads to distrust, poor teamwork, and decreased job performance — all of which compromise patient safety. A hospital's primary responsibility is to benefit and be accountable to the public it serves. However, when corporate leadership is allowed to eclipse cooperation and communication with antagonism and deception, it will undoubtedly destroy itself and those around it.

A typical hospital setting consists of a large group of professionals, paraprofessionals, and ancillary staff whose collective goal is to provide for the health, safety, and well-being of a given community. Although there is no stable and permanent subgroup in a society of chimpanzees, the same is not true in the healthcare setting — there are many stable and permanent subdivisions, especially in a hospital. These include business, financial, and IT departments as well as patient care areas such as the Emergency Department (ER or ED), Intensive Care Unit (ICU), Labor and Delivery (L&D), Surgery (OR), Recovery Room (PACU), and the Medical-Surgical (Med-Surg) floor or wards.

At this point, there are a couple of items that need highlighting. Healthcare workers are instructed to reference the Emergency Department as the ED, not the ER — the semantic rationale being that it is no longer a "room" but a department. This acronym can be confusing as the Education Department is also known as the ED (I once attended a seminar and identified my specialty by writing "ED" on my nametag; everyone thought my area of expertise was in education rather than emergency nursing). Therefore, out of respect for continuity and clarity for the general population, many providers still call the Emergency Department the ER.

In somewhat the same vein, many caregivers continue to call a person a patient, not a client (healthcare workers are told to use the term *client* instead of *patient*, which is notably one of many subtle corporate behavior modification tactics used to pervert an employee's beneficent conscience). A patient is a person who receives healthcare interventions, whereas a client is defined as a "consumer of a product, goods, or services." The term *patient* maintains a person's humanity. The word *client* is dehumanizing in that it depicts a customer who receives and pays for a product. By definition alone, the term *client* portrays an impersonal and indifferent business transaction that contradicts basic physician and nursing tenets.

In comparing primate and human communities, the chimp fusion-fission social subgroup is most similar to different nursing departments in that staff may temporarily be assigned, or 'float,' to another unit and later return to their base or home department. Some employees leave their unit by transferring to another area, while others may leave the employer completely by resigning their position. In either scenario, replacing the absentee employee is essential to the department's function and purpose, and the overall survival of the institution.

An open job position can create fierce competition especially for an experienced nurse, although age and professional experience are not always synonymous since a candidate's years of experience does not always equate to their chronological age. Consequently, an older person working in a skilled job or profession does not necessarily mean they have been doing it forever. In order to determine what number qualifies as "older," the U.S. federal government's Equal Employment Opportunity Commission (EEOC) quantifies age as a protected class of people who are 40 and older. Therefore, many older nurses may actually be recent (generally considered as 3 years or less) nursing school graduates who have yet to attain expertise.

Experienced nurses are often hard pressed to maintain or gain employment because they are near or at the top of the facility's pay scale. This holds true regardless whether a current staff member or seasoned applicant is union "protected," in an at-will facility (of which either the employee or employer can terminate employment, for any or no reason, without consequence), or a right-to-work state (in which employees are not required to be a union member or pay union dues). So if you see an older nurse during your next healthcare visit, they might be a relatively new nurse.

In addition to those workers lost to attrition, resignation, or termination, by 2020 nearly half of all American registered nurses will reach retirement age and the absence of talented nurses will be more than obvious to the healthcare consumer. To see the trending decline of experienced nurses all one has to do is look around their hospital or doctor's office to guesstimate nursing's median age. If experienced older nurses are becoming fewer and far between, then the million-dollar question is who is mentoring, precepting, and transitioning the new grads from theoretical to real-life practice?

Generally speaking, it's pretty much a sure bet that the novice nurse will be hired before the expert. After all, it does make better financial sense, and that's what healthcare is mostly about these days: profit before patients.

In an effort to maintain this 'money matters' mentality, rather than recruit qualified candidates who value a moral and ethical work culture and are seeking opportunity, advancement, and/or offer decades of experience, many triadic leaders pursue those who are most prone to obedience and conformity. Vacancies are often filled after painstaking interviews in order to find the "right fit"; while other times a warm body is better than no body and positions are filled with the next marginally qualified applicant. Neither rationale is ideal for the facility, nor for the health, safety, and well-being of the patients being served.

Those administrators and/or managers searching for the right fit are essentially recruiting like-minded narcissists, Machiavellians, and psychopaths that will perpetuate the corporation's cult mentality. Conversely, hiring a warm body is done in the hope of successfully programming and plugging that employee into the company's sociopathic work culture. In either case, the goal is to add another sycophant to the growing minion and mini-Mach population.

In both scenarios, the newbie will have their work cut out for them. As a new employee, regardless of age or experience, most people approach their new job with exhilarating anticipation and the hope for all things possible. Little do they know what they may be getting themselves into.

New Chimp

---

*"When it comes to controlling human
beings there is no better instrument than
lies. Because, you see, humans live by beliefs.
And beliefs can be manipulated."*

~ MICHAEL ENDE

TO THE FRESHLY HIRED, WHETHER a "new grad" or a seasoned professional, a facility orientation and department preceptor program is instrumental to an employee's success and long-term retention. Carmen Nobel, senior editor of *Working Knowledge* at Harvard Business School, explains:

> Employee orientation programs are much more successful when they are less about the company and more about the employee. The

first few minutes of new employee orientation, if done right, can lead to happier and more productive workers and, ultimately, increased customer satisfaction. Unfortunately, a lot of companies do it wrong.[30]

A corporation's disregard of the impact of a quality new employee orientation is tantamount to ignoring their profit-loss margin since it is well documented that frequent staff turnover can be extremely costly. It's been said that 'employees don't leave jobs, they leave managers.' And administrators manage managers.

In 2012, the United States Bureau of Labor Statistics reported, "for all positions except executive and physicians — jobs that require very specific skills — the typical (median) cost of turnover was 21 percent of an employee's annual salary. Jobs that are very complex and that require higher levels of education and specialized training tend to have even higher turnover costs." One of the many disturbing explanations for employee resignations is that "roughly 21 percent of nursing turnover can be related to incivility in the workplace" and this factor alone can cost up to $88,000 to replace just one nurse (American Nurses Association, 2015).

A company's orientation and department-specific preceptor program should serve to cultivate a partnership between the organization and employee in order to foster genuine employee commitment, and is fundamental to job satisfaction as well as the facility's solvency. New employee orientation is similar to a chimp community in that it provides an opportunity for the team to "exchange friendly greetings," and become acquainted with fellow employees and the corporate culture as a whole.

A typical orientation program begins with handing out company pens and travel mugs, and usually consists of two or three 8-hour days of classroom training conducted by speakers from various departments under the direction of a facilitator. The acclimation process traditionally starts with the corporation's mission, vision, and purpose presentation followed by a description of assorted employee programs and services the facility offers. Time is set aside for meet-and-greet and group activities that often include role-playing scenarios. Although orientation is generally considered a one-time event, it should be recognized as an ongoing process that serves to fortify employee and corporate success.

Once orientation is complete, the employee begins work in their department under the guidance of a preceptor. Preceptors serve to augment new hire orientation and cultivate successful job-role transition. This is the time when new employees become familiar with their area, and learn job-specific information necessary for individual, team, and department success which in turn may secure the company's longevity.

Anthropologist Dr. Dennis O'Neil's research illustrates how employee orientation is similar to primate socialization:

> When chimpanzee communities come together, they usually exchange friendly greetings rather than show aggression. However, it would be a mistake to assume from this that chimpanzee society is always peaceful. Often teamwork used to frighten and impress is more effective than any one individual's muscles in achieving chimpanzee goals.[31]

In the same manner, the ideal orientation often falls short in that many induction programs that appear to begin as a transformational employee process degenerate into the predetermined transactional employee behavior modification and integration system that actually fuels the organization. While transformational leadership allows the employee to perform their best without fear of reprisal, many organizations practice transactional leadership in order to achieve compliance and accomplish goals through a reward-punishment system.

Much of today's negative corporate culture could be avoided if companies would shift their focus from their own agenda to the employee by emphasizing the importance of the staff-member's role within the organization. Employee engagement can be established by merging the corporation's objectives with those of their employees. Staff motivation is accomplished through traditional (pay and compensation), emotional (personal growth), and professional (recognition and advancement) incentives. Additionally, because there is an inherent human tendency to form partnerships with those who share a common goal, it is important that staff understand the employer's expectations and the rationale of why they are required to perform a certain way.

One vital employment aspect rarely, if ever, presented during orientation is how the company acquires enough revenue to issue paychecks. A basic Economics 101 explanation of accounts payable and receivable might help employees realize exactly how essential they are to the organizational team. There are many factors that contribute to workplace conflict. Understanding the process of healthcare from a business perspective could allay one of the many 'them versus us' struggles, and just might incentivize employee engagement throughout the onboarding process.

Chimpanzees live in groups that demonstrate a "close association of young and old" through which "the young learn...from experienced, knowledgeable adults. The result is that by the time primates are grown, they are usually proficient in dealing with each other and the environment" (Dennis O'Neil, Ph.D., *Adaptations of Group Living*, n.d.). Just as young chimpanzees are shown the ropes by community elders, employers should gradually introduce their staff to some of the significant government influences that impact contemporary healthcare delivery systems.

In addition to previously discussed C-Mach, mini-Mach, and minion agendas, barriers to corporate success also include a plethora of financial challenges that result in additional conflict between healthcare professionals and the employer. To better understand the struggle between beneficence and business, a brief history is required to comprehend how a noble healthcare management endeavor more than 150 years ago, snowballed into the American financial fiasco it has become. Simply stated, healthcare reimbursement begins with the ICD.

Wikipedia explains:

The International Classification of Diseases (ICD) "is the international standard diagnostic tool for epidemiology, health management and clinical purposes [and] is maintained [and published] by the World Health Organization (WHO). The beginning of the ICD dates back to 1860 when Florence Nightingale made a proposal that was to result in the development of the first model of [a] systemic collection of hospital data. [Several decades later], French physician Jacques Bertillon introduced the *Bertillon Classification of Causes of Death*. In 1898, the American Public Health Association (APHA) recommended that the registrars of Canada, Mexico, and the United States…adopt it and suggested it be revised every ten years. In 1948, the World Health Organization (WHO) assumed responsibility for preparing and publishing the [periodic] revisions, and the existing United States ICD came into being nearly 60 years ago. Currently, "the ICD is used by physicians, researchers, health information managers and coders, [as well as] insurers and patient organizations to classify diseases and other health problems recorded on many types of health and vital records, including death certificates. These records also provide the basis for the compilation of national mortality and morbidity statistics by WHO Member States. Finally, [the] ICD is used for reimbursement."[32]

After the ICD-9 completed its tenth revision, full compliance of the ICD-10 began October 1, 2015. However, University of Illinois at Chicago (UIC) Associate Director of Public Affairs Jeanne Galatzer-Levy (2015) reports that UIC warned of serious deficiencies months before the October ICD-10 implementation:

> Emergency medicine faces special challenges during this fall's changeover in how medical diagnoses are coded. Nearly a quarter of all ER clinical encounters could pose difficulties. In addition to the problems it may pose for reimbursement and proper clinical documentation, the coding change will complicate tasks…such as justifying hospital admissions. [UIC researchers] found that 27 percent of the 1,830 commonly used emergency room ICD-9 codes had convoluted mappings that could create problems with reporting or reimbursement. Further, they found that when they looked at more than 24,000 actual clinical

encounters in the ER, 23 percent could be assigned incorrect codes if recommendations of the CMS were followed. The ICD-10 includes more than 68,000 diagnostic codes — compared to 14,000 in its predecessor, ICD-9.

To make business matters more challenging for healthcare providers, less than two years after the ICD-10's release, ICD-11 compliance is earmarked for 2017.

Simply put, the ICD is a disease, illness, and injury classification system based on "a wide variety of signs, symptoms, abnormal findings, complaints, social circumstances, and external causes of injury or disease" (ibid,[32]). In addition to its global use for morbidity and mortality statistics, the ICD establishes the criteria on which medical healthcare reimbursement is determined.

However superfluous it may seem, it is important to mention the ICD's analogous counterpart, the Diagnostic and Statistical Manual of Mental Disorders (DSM). Although the DSM spectrum is limited to mental and behavioral conditions, the common denominator between the ICD and DSM is that each one respectively classifies medical and mental health disorders, and provides diagnostic and decision support — all of which determine reimbursement. Healthcare has long segregated mental from physical health making the DSM fundamentally irrelevant to medical reimbursement. However, because of collaborative agreements between the two agencies, mental healthcare reimbursement is achieved through "crosswalks" that bridge DSM diagnostic codes with ICD codes.

Healthcare reimbursement is based on billing codes that standardize descriptions of the patient's illness, injury, and procedures described through the International Classification of Diseases (ICD), the Diagnostic and Statistical Manual of Mental Disorders (DSM), and Current Procedural Terminology (CPT). CPT is a numerical code set that identifies medical procedures and "services rendered rather than the diagnosis" (Wikipedia, 2015). Services rendered include ambulance transports, medical equipment, and supplies. Healthcare providers list these codes on billing records and often within the medical records themselves.

The advent of the electronic medical record (EMR) ushered in the digital version of the hand-written patient paper chart. EMRs were designed to electronically document a patient's diagnosis and treatment and, like the paper chart, are used solely within the clinician's practice, office, or hospital department(s). And like the paper chart, an EMR cannot be disseminated to or accessed by anyone outside the immediate patient care environment except by physically (versus digitally) delivering the needed data. Freelance health reporter Eric Whitney describes one of the many EMR challenges:

> Technology entrepreneur Jonathan Bush says he was recently watching a patient move from a hospital to a nursing home. The patient's information was in an electronic medical record, or EMR. And getting the patient's records from the hospital to the nursing home, Bush says, wasn't exactly a drag and drop.
> "These two guys then type — I kid you not — the printout from the brand new EMR into *their* EMR, so that their fax server can fax it to the bloody nursing home," Bush says. US taxpayers have poured $30 billion into funding electronic records systems in hospitals and doctors' offices since 2009. But most of those systems still can't talk to each other, which makes transfer of medical information tough (NPR, March 2015).

Although the terms EMR and EHR (electronic health record) are often used interchangeably, the National Alliance for Health Information Technology (NAHIT) differentiates the two acronyms:

EMR: the electronic record of health-related information on an individual that is created, gathered, managed, and consulted by licensed clinicians and staff *from a single organization* who are involved in the individual's health and care.

EHR: the aggregate electronic record of health-related information on an individual that is created and gathered cumulatively *across more than one health care organization* and is managed and consulted by licensed clinicians and staff involved in the individual's health and care. By these definitions, an EHR is an EMR with [nationally recognized] interoperability [standards] (i.e. integration to other providers' systems) (Neal, 2008).

The EMR is a limited medical record management system within one organization whereas the EHR includes the medical record as well as specific features for billing and management purposes across a spectrum of health delivery systems. The EHR allows billing codes to be directly pulled and readily verified through clinician documentation. If practices cannot validate a charge, they should not bill for it (if it isn't documented it wasn't done, and billing for an undocumented intervention is fraud).

Early EMR/EHR users quickly realized that electronic documentation is primarily a billing program that ineffectively records all-things patients including interventions, course of treatment, and care. Outward appearances suggest the EHR offers a complete and comprehensive medical record and electronic billing system in one efficient data package. However, practitioners who use these systems have direct knowledge of its underlying purpose: it is an individualized patient billing program generated by ticking pre-determined patient assessment, treatment, and evaluation boxes. Free-text caregiver notes are discouraged by design, and are a limited option in many EHR systems.

The emergence of the EMR/EHR is a direct result of the economic stimulus package called the American Recovery and Reinvestment Act (ARRA) that was signed into law on February 17, 2009 by President Obama. A provision of this Recovery Act required the adoption of electronic medical records (EMRs) by 2014. According to the U.S. Department of Health and Human Services, the ARRA "authorizes the CMS to provide a reimbursement incentive for physician and hospital providers who are successful in becoming "meaningful users" of an electronic health record (EHR)." Incentive payments began in 2011 "and gradually phase[d] down. Starting in 2015, providers are expected to have adopted and be actively utilizing an EHR in compliance with the "meaningful use" definition or they will be subject to financial penalties under Medicare." Non-compliant providers "will experience a 1% penalty reduction in Medicare reimbursements, and rates of reduction will likely rise annually thereafter" (USF Health, 2013).

In addition to accurate ICD, DSM, and CPT diagnostic coding and supportive documentation requirements, it must be remembered that the Centers for Medicare and Medicaid Services (CMS) — formerly known as the Health Care Financing Administration (HCFA) until its name changed in 2001 — accounts for 90% of hospital and healthcare financial reimbursement. Under the CMS umbrella, a large part of reimbursement is also determined by yet another federal healthcare requirement: patient satisfaction scores. The Department of Health and Human Services (HHS), which oversees the CMS, explains that "hospitals are no longer paid solely based on the quantity of services they provide. CMS rewards hospitals based on the quality of care provided to Medicare patients… The Hospital Value-Based Purchasing Program (VBP) was "established under the Affordable Care Act of 2010 [and] makes incentive payments to hospitals based…on an approved set of measures and dimensions grouped into specific quality domains."[33]

While Medicare pays for hospital provided services, its focus is on Value-Based Purchasing quality hospital service. Since 30% of a hospital's Medicare reimbursement is based on patient satisfaction survey scores alone, failure to meet VBP guidelines guarantees stiff monetary penalties in the form of reimbursement reductions, and threatens the institution's very survival. Organizations, left with virtually no choice, are shifting their focus from a fee-for-service (quantity) schedule toward VBP (quality) models of care.

Freelance health writer Debra Wood, RN (*Nurse-Patient Communication Affects Hospital Consumer Metrics*, 2013) clarifies one of many VBP "quality domains" — nursing communication:

> The CMS will determine 30 percent of hospital's VBP incentive payments by how patients evaluate their stay... Improving nurse-patient communication could result in gains in other Hospital Consumer Assessment of Healthcare Providers and Systems (HCAHPS) metrics, including responsiveness of hospital staff, pain management, communication about medication and overall patient experience scores, which together affect 15 percent of hospitals' value-based purchasing (VBP) incentive payments, according to a new study

released by Press Ganey Associates... [Press Ganey is] a patient experience improvement firm."[34]

In 2011 the CMS announced "that patient satisfaction survey results will be one significant factor in determining Medicare reimbursements, and for those executives lucky enough to meet the contrived guidelines, bonuses. [Additionally]...patient satisfaction surveys were fully integrated into the 2010 Affordable Care Act, through healthcare quality measures" (DeMoro, *National Nurses United*, 2012).

The impetus for what appears to be corporate collusion can be strongly attributed to the external monetary demands and incentives guided by performance metric entities (patient satisfaction scorekeepers) such as Press Ganey and HCAHPS.

According to the University of Illinois at Chicago (2009):

Desperate to meet these initiatives, healthcare organizations attempt to increase patient and satisfaction scores by utilizing marketing companies. One such healthcare marketing company, the Studer Group, is widely utilized to positively boost patient flow, corporate profit, and name-branding.

In her 2012 blog, National Nurses United executive director RoseAnn DeMoro describes how "nursing scripts and patient satisfaction surveys project a fantasy of care, not real care. This deception includes "scripts" and "rounding" guidelines provided by exorbitantly paid consultants like the Studer Group and Press Ganey. Strict adherence to scripts for every RN-patient interaction is quickly becoming a job expectation. Since RN non-compliance can lead to decreased Medicare reimbursement, failure to meet these requirements can lead to reprimand or other forms of discipline including termination." Of the many elements within the Studer Group package, AIDET® is the ground zero employee behavior modification strategy used to improve patient satisfaction scores. AIDET is an acronym that represents the *Five Fundamentals of Service*: **A**cknowledge, **I**ntroduce, **D**uration, **E**xplanation, and **T**hank You.

According to Studer, "Organizations who have hardwired the Five Fundamentals of Service through consistent use by all employees find this practice correlates closely with high patient satisfaction. After you've introduced AIDET to staff, hardwire it. Ask department leaders to complete an AIDET competency checklist as they round on their employees to see who's consistently using [AIDET]. Finally, give pop quizzes! 'You'd be surprised how well you can align the world around chocolate,' says [Studer Group Senior Coach] Don Dean who gives out chocolate bars to staff who get it right."[35]

The Studer Group stresses the importance of AIDET because "global ratings of care are more closely linked to communication than technical skill, [it improves] quality outcomes, affects reimbursement to hospitals, reduces malpractice and complaint events [and it is the] primary driver to attain and retain patients. [And remember to] manage-up other members of the care team [to] improve patient perception..."[36]

There are many challenges in a structured "customer service" system within a healthcare setting. Examples of how Studer and Studeresque theories translate into real-life clinical practice include these employee observations:

* "The problem with Studer…is the principles were never fully adhered to. Admin would pick and choose certain areas of Studer to use, and ignore the rest. No program will work effectively if the entire program is not implemented and reinforced consistently. What should be more worrisome is the upcoming ICD-10 implementation and the ill prepared hospital that is far from ready for this massive change. With little to no cash on hand how will [hospitals]

survive this transition that effects [sic] all billing from all areas of the hospital and clinics?"

- "Caregivers have said that while they were trying to do their work with patients, a person would be looking over their shoulder to assure that the AIDET mantra was being precisely followed. One nurse noted that she was expected to gush to the patient that the patient was so fortunate to have [so-and-so] as his doctor, as he was exceptionally talented. She felt she was being asked to be a salesperson rather than a caregiver."

- "The problem I had with the structured AIDET approach is that it totally depersonalized my patient interactions. When I deal with a patient, what I tell them and how I say it depends on age, situation, condition, and even the time of day. There is a time to say I have 30 plus years of experience, and there is a time to simply listen and show empathy. But with AIDET, you had to give the script every time, and yes, you had someone with a clipboard listening and recording [employee compliance with AIDET during patient encounters]. The patient actually became secondary to the process."[37]

As hospitals strive to comply with the Value-Based Purchasing (VBP) demands, employers insist that customer service scripts be adhered to first and foremost. Both VBP and employers dismiss the selfless foundation of medicine and nursing by creating a popularity contest upon which the hospitals' very existence depends. Although these financial incentives may be perceived as unethical, immoral, and detrimental to the health, safety, and well-being of all who seek medical care in the United States, the federal government is forcing healthcare institutions and workers to sacrifice patients for profit.

When push comes to shove, doing the right thing often overrides doing things the right way. Reciting AIDET and other "fantasies of care" should be disregarded when patients' lives hang in the balance. Healthcare professionals are expected to demonstrate clinical competence, expertise, and compassion. Adept caregivers integrate their professional moral commitment to the well-being of others, and strive to provide the best care to patients, all while respecting the individuals' healthcare needs and goals. Serving patients during illness, injury, and disease, and supporting their health during times of wellness, is as fundamental to nursing as are technical skills.

Most people understand that customer service "is the provision of service to customers before, during and after a purchase"[38] and is a profession in and of itself. It is a specific career track with its own professional organizations such as the International Customer Service Association (ICSA) and National Customer Service Association (NCSA). The ICSA even offers a certification program that serves "to advance, strengthen, and promote the industry of Professional Customer Service [and] assist individuals and organizations with their professional growth, development, and recognition..." (ICSA, 2015).

The *Atlantic* article, "The Problem with Satisfied Patients," explains the dangers of hospital customer service incentives:

> The Centers for Medicare and Medicaid Services officials wrote "Delivery of high-quality, patient-centered care requires us to carefully consider the patient's experience in the hospital inpatient setting." They probably had no idea that their methods could end up indirectly harming patients...A misguided attempt to improve healthcare has led some hospitals to focus on making people happy, rather than making them well" (Robbins, 2015).

Quality healthcare is defined as "safe, effective, patient-centered, timely, efficient and equitable" (Institute of Medicine, 2001) and "as doing the right thing for the right patient, at the right time, in the right way to achieve the best possible results" (Agency for Healthcare Research and Quality, n.d.). Although VBP was written as a "quality" metric reimbursement guide, it has nothing to do with medical care; it is exclusively a patient satisfaction scorecard. The CMS and hospitals continue to disregard standards of quality medical care by demanding quality hospital marketing. A high ranking on the Press-Ganey satisfaction scorecard equates to "generous and hospitable treatment of guests or customers of an organization,"[39] not professional expertise, competency, or quality of medical intervention(s). VBP holds "hospitals accountable for patient perceptions."[40]

All of which brings us back to the employee orientation process and its importance in acclimating new, as well as existing, employees to the often-changing government demands of a healthcare entity's fiscal accountability and compliance. In order to sustain a viable healthcare center, the employer must develop skilled and committed employees who are not only competent, but are a "company man." Author Cynthia Shapiro, a former HR executive, cautions, "You must outwardly act like you support the company's policies and interests no matter what you really think" (*Corporate Confidential*, 2005). Even the marginally capable employee helps the facility's profitability by doing whatever the company dictates in order to ensure everyone has a roof over their heads.

Just as our chimp cousin's primary predatory threat is habitat destruction and disease, so it is in the healthcare community. As current federal and corporate mandates stand, if citizens and healthcare workers do not learn to adapt to the influences of government predators, illness, injury, and disease will run rampant as our hospitals become non-existent.

Americans who want to keep their preferred doctor and hospital in business will have to fill out those satisfaction surveys; making sure they give top scores in all categories or it doesn't count. It wouldn't be surprising if someday the CMS demands that patients fill out satisfaction surveys with the understanding that non-compliance will result in non-coverage of provider visits.

Present circumstances require healthcare workers, above all else, keep patients happy, with health and well-being a secondary goal. Until the American government's healthcare financial incentive clause is amended or eliminated, employees will be expected to obey their employers' dictates or suffer the consequences. It is up to health professionals to find a balance between best clinical practice and customer service representative functions in order to circumvent severe reprimand up to and including termination. However, if the government and transactional healthcare organizations continue to sacrifice patients for profit (not to mention C-Mach, mini-Mach, and minion agendas) there will forever be workplace conflict.

As in the chimp world where teamwork is "used to frighten and impress [in achieving] goals," so it is in the majority of today's healthcare environment. Both new and established employees often find themselves in the position of having to choose sides. Most find it safer to join the status quo and become one of the bullies rather than be bullied. Is it as simple as, "if you can't beat 'em, join 'em," or is there a primordial motivation that perpetuates the human culture of intimidation?

Bad Chimp

"Employers control the work environment. Good employers purge bullies, most promote them."

~ GARY NAMIE, PH.D.

WHERE DO BULLIES COME FROM? Is it genetic? Taught? Environmental? Nature or nurture? None, some, or all of the above? Perhaps it's simply the primitive instinct that, in most people, lies dormant in the recesses of our reptilian brain. No matter the theory, "conspecific [same species] aggression is intended to increase the social dominance of the organism relative to the dominance position of other organisms" (Ferguson & Beaver, 2009).

Biopsychologist and behavioral neuroscientist Alice G. Walton, Ph.D. (*Forbes*, July 5, 2012) explains:

In the most basic terms, bullying is about dominating — and we come from ancestors who were big into the dominance hierarchy. As Christopher Boehm, Ph.D., who literally wrote the book on it (*Moral Origins*), says, "Any species that has a social dominance hierarchy, like apes or monkeys…has bullies." He adds that bullying is adaptive for many species… "because you get better food or mating opportunities… In primates, studies have shown that the top bullies have more offspring and therefore their genes proliferate." So there's a clear payoff to it, since the more you bully, the higher you'll rise in social ranks… Ancient parts of our brains still exist, and inform our behavior in lots of maladaptive ways. Bullying is a great example of this.[41]

It is evident that our ancestral "daily battle for survival has now transferred to the workplace" (Field, 1996). British anti-bullying activist Tim Field observed that "bullying consists of the least competent most aggressive employee projecting their incompetence on to the least aggressive most competent employee and winning" (*Bully in Sight*, 1996). This statement is supported through current publications based on contemporary studies and research. The general consensus is that unbridled hostility can result in systematic workplace terrorism commonly referred to as bullying.

In 2010, the University of Louisville reported that "roughly one-fourth of employed Americans have reported bullying at work. That's over 30 million people."

Current statistics reveal that:

"According to David Maxfield, coauthor of the books *Crucial Conversations* and *Influencer*, 96% of American employees experience bullying in the workplace, and the nature of that bullying is changing. 89% of those bullies have been at it for more than a year...54% have been bullying for more than five years... [and] 80% of bullies affect five or more people." One of the statistics that was most shocking to Maxfield was the multiple forms bullying took. The study looked at three categories: sabotaging of others' work or reputations; browbeating, threats, or intimidation; and physical intimidation or assault. "Another stat that really surprised me: how long it's gone on," says Maxfield. "You would think it would be intolerable."[42]

Bullying is an element of social psychology in which behaviors are manipulated, rather than influenced, by those who control the environment. Mini-Machs and minions demonstrate intimidation and aggression in which "the behavior is intended to harm or disturb...occurs repeated[ly] over time and there is an imbalance of power with a more powerful person or group attacking a less powerful one. This asymmetry of power may be physical or psychological, and the aggressive behavior may be verbal (e.g. name-calling, threats), physical (e.g. hitting), or psychological (e.g. rumors, shunning, exclusion). The key elements of this definition are that multiple means can be employed by the bully or bullies, intimidation is the goal, and bullying can happen on a one-on-one or group basis" (Nansel et al., 2001).

Bullying is one of several forms of workplace violence (WPV), and any form of repeated intimidation and aggression used to modify another person's behavior qualifies as such. As arbitrator Bernice Fields, J.D. explains, "Violence in the workplace begins long before fists fly or lethal weapons extinguish lives. Where resentment and aggression routinely displace cooperation and communication, violence has occurred."

The World Health Organization (WHO) defines workplace violence as:

> Incidents where staff are abused, threatened or assaulted in circumstances related to their work...involving an explicit or implicit challenge to their safety, well-being or health... Psychological violence is currently emerging as a priority concern at the workplace [and is the] intentional use of power...against another person or group, that can result in harm to physical, mental, spiritual, moral, or social development. It includes verbal abuse, bullying/mobbing, harassment and threats.[43]

To understand what external influences activate our reptilian-brain instinct to intimidate others, a look at environmental factors is required. Most of us are familiar with the traditional childhood terms *bully* and *victim*. While we know that a victim is the recipient of a bully's aggression, writer and biological anthropologist Dr. Gwen Dewar defines two distinct categories of bullies:

> Kids who harass and intimidate others were once lumped together. But today, researchers have identified two different types of bully. The "pure" bullies are the confident aggressors. They dish out intimidation and harassment. In general, they don't get victimized by

other bullies. The "bully-victims," by contrast, are both bullies and the victims of bullying.[44]

Pure bullies "always occupy the dominant role. They don't get victimized by other bullies. They are at the top of the food chain. And they seem to reap the benefits of their position."[45] Bully-victims are those who have been bullied and eventually become bullies themselves.

Bullying is a cycle of abuse that often comes from a long lineage that is handed down from parent to child; it is a multigenerational transmission process through which actions, reactions, and behaviors are programmed. Parents model verbal and non-verbal behaviors that communicate what they consider acceptable and normal. And children say what they hear and do what they see.

Parental bully-modeling includes verbal, physical, and emotional abuse.

- Verbal abuse, such as name calling (a parent belittles another person's appearance, personality, or disability), identifies targets based on the way they look, act, or behave.
- Physical abuse employs brute actions to gain and maintain power and control over their child.

- Emotional abuse is defined as covert relational passive-aggressive actions, often mingled between acts of generosity, which serve to break a child's confidence and self-esteem, and parent-child trust.

Educational psychologist Dr. Sonia Sharp explains that "humans have taken an ancient behavior that used to provide an advantage in survival and reproduction and altered its intensity and impact through language and culture. While physical bullying is a serious issue and targets of bullying are beaten all too often, humans have intensified and expanded the impact of bullying by incorporating language. [Verbal and nonverbal] language allows us to communicate abstract ideas, coordinate behaviors and express thoughts and feelings to others."[46]

The child who learns how to bully from a parent may eventually become adept at intimidating those who are perceived as some sort of threat, regardless whether that threat is real or imagined. Additionally, living in violent neighborhoods often prompts parents to intentionally teach their children to attack others that "may include kicking, hitting, or taking a victim's personal belongings"[47] — rationalizing that the best defense is a better offense. Health and labor economist Anna Aizer, Ph.D. observes that "three quarters of American children have been exposed to neighborhood violence in their lifetimes. Most of the existing research has concluded that exposure to violence leads to...aggressive behavior" (ibid,[47]).

Children who have been bullied themselves who go on to bully others are called bully-victims. It's been observed that, "Just as abusive parents often were abused as children, bullying has a cycle of repetition where the victim becomes a bully."[48] Wayne Parsons, J.D. confirms that "a recent study of bullying in JAMA Psychiatry (*Adult Psychiatric Outcomes of Bullying and Being Bullied by Peers in Childhood and Adolescence*, 2013) shows conclusive evidence that a bullied child often becomes a bully to someone else."[49]

Because over "90%, of the nearly 3.5 million nurses nationwide, are female" (Bureau of Health Professions, National Center for Health Workforce Analysis, April, 2013), a significant portion of nursing's workplace bullies are women. Human behavior, parenting, and education expert Dr. Gail Gross explains:

> The female bully is "often...someone who is bullied or abused at home and, feeling out of control, imposes her will over others, modeling the behavior of her own family network. Further, bullying behavior reflects an immaturity in both coping skills and social

interactions, with a lack of empathy as a defining characteristic. Moreover, bullies reach back towards an earlier stage of development where their needs were met narcissistically" (Huffington Post, *Girls Who Bully and the Women They Learn From*, January 23, 2014).

These women have little to no control over their home life, and often find respite in controlling others in the workplace. They are the peers and superiors who experience a taste of confidence, self-esteem, and human worth through intimidation and bullying. Work is the place where they believe they can control their life and claim their turn at empowerment.

Bullying Statistics (2015) explains:

One would think that as people mature and progress through life, that they would stop behaviors of their youth. Unfortunately, this is not always the case. Sadly, adults can be bullies, just as children and teenagers can be bullies. While adults are more likely to use verbal bullying as opposed to physical bullying, the fact of the matter is that adult bullying exists. The goal of an adult bully is to gain power over another person, and make himself or herself the dominant adult. They try to humiliate victims, and "show them who is boss."[50]

Power gives one the authority to direct and influence the behavior of others. Bullies use this power to intimidate and manipulate another's behavior by homing in on the targets' vulnerabilities. Author Amy Tan observes, "You see what power is — holding someone else's fear in your hand and showing it to them."

Regardless of their origin, bullies harbor deep-seated insecurities, and have no compunction exploiting someone else's real or contrived imperfections. They attempt to compensate for their perceived personal failures by convincing themselves of (or attempt to establish) their professional worth at the expense of their peers and subordinates.

Having glimpsed into the origins of bullying, we now have a better understanding of where bullies come from, and may even feel empathetic toward their genesis. However, pangs of compassion should in no way excuse or absolve the life-altering and traumatic long-term effect of their behavior.

Sad Chimp

---

*"Here is the tragedy: when you are the victim...
not only do you feel utterly helpless and abandoned
by the world, you also know that very few people
can understand, or even begin to believe, that
life can be this painful. There is nothing I can
think of that is quite as isolating as this"*

~ GILES ANDREAE

THE EFFECT BULLYING HAS ON its target creates incomprehensible devastation. If you have never been a victim of bullying then it is nearly impossible to describe the target's overwhelming mind, body, and spiritual fragmentation. Victims are made to feel incompetent, inconsequential, and useless. One of the workplace bully's many goals is to convince vetted co-workers and/or subordinates that they serve no purpose to anyone, including themselves, whereby victims are frequently driven to question their very existence.

Having spent many years witnessing and personally experiencing all of the above, I have come to realize that all hope is not lost. Understanding the bully's mindset, motives, and endgame is imperative not only to victim survival, but for personal and professional success. The steps to transitioning from victim to survivor begin with the ability to identify bullying behavior, recognizing the bully, and understanding the effects of abuse — and then doing something about it.

Researchers describe domineering chimpanzee behavior as an attempt "to intimidate a subordinate or to gain rank [by] standing up straight with hair bristling, shoulders hunched, and a compressed lips face so that his body looks larger and his face meaner."[51] Since human bullying body language is not usually as obvious, the first step to addressing intimidating behavior is recognizing the signs that there is a bully among us.

Bullies have a knack for studying their target, recognizing even a remote hint of vulnerability, and they possess a patient reserve in developing calculated attacks. They have an uncanny ability to sum up a victim's weaknesses, then strike when the target least expects it. Identifying bullying behavior is one of the first steps toward successfully deflecting the premeditated fear and intimidation that is workplace terrorism.

Often the bully's endgame includes the company's perverted strategy to methodically process an employee out of a job. To avoid becoming a victim, targets must first recognize the cues that they are earmarked for removal. In her book, *Corporate Confidential* (2005), Cynthia Shapiro outlines seven "danger signs" that "you might be in the process of being managed out":

1. You're feeling grossly ignored, overworked, underpaid, or set up to be unsuccessful.
2. Your boss doesn't seem to like you or pay attention to you the way he does to others.
3. Your office is moved to an undesirable location or you are regularly given the assignments no one else wants.
4. You're being given impossible tasks with unrealistic deadlines.
5. Your boss surprises you with a scathing performance review.
6. The company brings in someone to "help" you with your work and you find yourself training her in the nuances of your position and tasks.
7. Your company moves you from department to department so you never have a chance to complete anything.

In addition to these seven danger signs, the target may concurrently experience the psychosocial effects of bullying. Health and fitness journalist Allison Van Dusen (*Forbes*, 2008) accurately categorizes the "Ten Signs You're Being Bullied at Work":

1. Work Means Misery: If you often feel like throwing up or are particularly anxious the night before the start of your workweek, there's a good chance you're experiencing workplace bullying, experts say. While few people look forward to Mondays, they shouldn't cause you to feel physically ill.
2. Constant Criticism: If the criticism from your boss or co-worker never seems to stop, despite your history of objective competence and even excellence, a bully might be to blame. Workplace bullies also tend to have a different standard in mind for their targets, experts say.
3. Lots of Yelling: Overt workplace bullies tend to make their feelings known by yelling. If you are frequently screamed at, insulted, or humiliated in front of others, you're probably being bullied.
4. Remembering Your Mistakes: If your boss or co-worker seems to keep a file of your mistakes [which they do] and constantly refer to them

for no constructive reason [which they will], you're likely being bullied. Falsely accusing you of errors is another common tactic.
5. Gossip and Lies: A covert office bully is more likely to spread destructive gossip and lies about you and your performance, rather than scream at you in front of your co-workers. Failing to stop the spread of a rumor can be an act of bullying, too.
6. You're Not Invited to Lunch or Meetings: If you feel like you're being singled out and/or isolated by your co-workers or boss, socially or physically, you are probably being bullied, experts say. That can mean having your desk moved or not being invited to meetings or even lunch.
7. You Always Need Mental Health Days: If it seems like all of your paid time off is being used for mental health breaks or to get away from the misery of your office, it could be because you're being bullied. Other signs include spending your days off feeling lifeless or your family members showing frustration over your constant obsessing about work.
8. Sabotage: A workplace bully may try to find ways to ensure that you fail at your job. Examples include changing rules on the fly

that apply to your work or not performing tasks crucial to your success, such as signing off on details or taking calls.
9. Impossible Schedule: A workplace bully won't hesitate to change your schedule to make your life more difficult. If your boss always schedules last minute late meeting on the days when he knows you're taking night classes or you have to pick up the kids, for instance, he or she may be a bully.
10. Stolen Work: You've been working day and night for weeks on a project that's now getting a good buzz at your office. If your boss or co-worker steals the credit, and has a habit of doing so, you're being bullied.

No matter your job, these seventeen indicators can be modified to fit any profession. Although it may take some time for the target, as well as bystanders, to recognize the often-subtle signs of bullying, it must be remembered that bullying is repeated, unwanted behavior toward another person or group of persons, and it can be perpetrated by one person or a group of people. Bullying can take the form of behaviors that include condescending language, lack of vital communication, unfair or inequitable work assignments and tasks, lack of teamwork (in which you're left to inevitably sink), retaliation, unwarranted criticisms, and undermining one's ability or competence.

The US Census Bureau reports that male nurses make up only about 9% of America's 3.5 million nurses (2013). Since 91% of nurses are predominantly women, overt bullying is fairly easy to recognize. Many of these women are the mean girls "who believe the world belongs to them and them only. They gossip about anyone that stands up to them and try to ruin their life."[54] Mean girls display their lack of emotional intelligence by avoiding responsibility and accountability as they empower themselves by diminishing the reputation of others.

Their technique is obvious and predictable as mean girls tend to 'tag-team' one person, often within a specific group of people, one month then switch to another person for another month, and on down the line until the first target is back up for grabs. It's a never-ending cycle of workplace harassment and incivility that, although annoying, is relatively harmless — unless they are purposed scouts who vet targets and then report back to their department mini-Mach and/or C-Machs.

Most workplace bullies are not usually as obvious in their calculated, self-serving agenda. To recognize the bully, we must be aware that sometimes the bully will make it clear that they don't like you right off the bat, while at other times the bully may befriend you by gaining your trust and making you think you are part of the team — until they throw you under the bus. Bullies will also repeatedly ostracize their victim by making it clear the target is not welcome in 'their' group. Unwitting targets find themselves being professionally isolated until they realize that they have been shunned, and are not welcome. Bullies publicly and privately harass, humiliate, and embarrass their target as their deliberate emotional deconstruction slowly reduces the employee to an unrecognizable shadow of the successful and respected colleague they once were.

The effect of workplace bullying can be devastating to the victims' emotional, psychological, physical, and mental health. Recalling my own egregious experience with a bully-boss, I now recognize that my habit of always giving the benefit of the doubt was actually a non-confrontational tendency to excuse bad behavior. Consequently, it took about four years to realize that I had been targeted, and by that time I was already showing signs of victimization.

The attacks were insidious and innocent appearing at first, until I noticed that I could set my calendar to every three weeks by predicting when the confrontations would occur. I recall trying to figure out what was happening when, alone in my kitchen one day, I stopped dead in my tracks as the thought came to me that maybe I was being bullied. I had never personally been bullied or a victim of this kind of fear and intimidation, and I was stunned. As I tried to process this revelation, I began to search everything I could to find out about adult bullying, workplace violence, and what to do about it.

During my research, I found myself traversing through Elizabeth Kubler-Ross' grief cycle model, "The Five Stages of Grief" (*On Death and Dying*, 1969). My reaction began with the denial stage; I was shocked, in disbelief, and unsure if my epiphany was correct. I tried my best to ignore this was happening until further research and studying convinced me otherwise. Once I was certain I had been targeted, my denial turned rather quickly to the anger phase. Thoughts such as "how dare they!" and "why are they doing this?" became my obsession for many months, which gradually stretched into several years. My anger vacillated between denial (not wanting to deal with this), to paranoia, anxiety, confusion, insomnia, agoraphobia, and depression, all of which became so intense that I would become physically ill. Anxiety tremors, headaches, stomach pain, and nausea became my new normal.

The bucolic island community in which I live used to be the playground for my joy of life. That quickly transformed into an unsafe place where uncertainty and perceived threats lurked around every corner. I retreated to our home where the shades were always drawn and lights were dimmed to create a safe-haven for my unraveling psyche.

During my scheduled 12-hour work nights, I found myself slipping into a sleep-work cycle that would become a sleep-sleep cycle on my days off. If I had to go out of the house for anything, I did so with palpable trepidation and anxiety. As the bullying became more overt, my world became smaller. I was afraid to say or do anything for fear of making things worse for myself. My focus narrowed to only work-related topics; all I did was sleep, eat, and breathe work. I had no interest in the world around me, including my family, unless it was about work. My confusion and panic led me on an obsession-fueled emotional rollercoaster of searching for answers that I hoped would make sense of what was happening. I simply could not understand how someone who took an oath of benevolence could be so heartless, disengaged, and downright mean to another colleague. I thought we nurses were all in this together. I thought we were a team with the collective purpose of empowering others — patients and colleagues alike — to feel better about themselves, and helping them achieve and maintain a state of well-being. Try as I might, I just didn't get it.

While I strived to advance my vocation, administration was pushing me to the back of the professional queue. Retrospectively, during my last six years of employment someone somewhere wanted me gone. Some of the administratively selected colleagues, peers and physicians confided in me that they were told to "monitor" my every move and report back to the Chief Nursing Officer. At one point, I was physically micromanaged for several weeks by the CNO themself as they hovered over me while I performed my bedside patient-care duties. When they couldn't find fault with my nursing knowledge, clinical skills or competency, they began to call random one-on-one meetings that were of no meaningful consequence, and my schedule was changed to the point that it looked like I was a new grad again with no rhyme, reason, or rhythm to my days off or on; it was as inconsistent as they come.

The improprieties imposed upon me by nursing's C-Mach, mini-Machs and their minions are too numerous to mention individually, however I will say they ranged from petty, non-consequential comments to significant defamatory lies. There were times when they pushed their contrived allegations of standards of practice deviations very hard. I invalidated their claims by presenting relevant state statutes; nursing codes of ethics, practice, and conduct; evidence-based practice (EBP) models; federal healthcare directives; and hospital policies that supported my clinical decision making process. They could not legitimately refute state, federal, or even their own corporate mandates. If the situation called for a more personal 'defense,' I presented hard-copies of applicable paper trails such as e-mails, awards, and letters of commendation from peers, colleagues, patients, and past bosses that I had received throughout my tenure. My current superiors had nothing concrete to disprove the tangible truth other than unsubstantiated "he said, she said" recounts.

Since they couldn't 'get me' on any standard of practice or hospital rule violations, the punishment came through other means such as:

- When I submitted a three-month advance request for two days off to celebrate a milestone wedding anniversary, it was denied with no valid reason provided.
- I received sporadic, abrupt, and inequitable schedule changes.
- I was required to attend 'last minute' mandatory one-on-one meetings with my superior(s) scheduled in the middle of my workday sleep-time.

- I was denied time off to receive an award at the hospital's annual employee recognition ceremony.

Then there was the day, after serving as the shift charge nurse for many years, I was suddenly, without warning or notification, deleted from that position. When I asked about this abrupt change, the manager told me that I was "getting old, [I] wouldn't be around much longer, and we need to get the younger nurses trained because they'll be the ones taking care of [me] soon…" (all of which was overheard by another seasoned RN who was passing by the open office door). It was one of those employee nightmares many of us have heard about but never thought was real.

There are many more examples, however, the most flagrant retaliatory action came around the time I filed an EEOC protected class discrimination complaint. One busy ER night, while working two RN staff members short, I had a mental health patient who escalated to the point of being a danger to self and others, and needed to be restrained for everyone's protection. In an ideal environment, it is recommended that five people assist in '4-pointing' a patient, with no less than a four staff-assist being acceptable. However, the ER is not always a perfect situation — especially when the department is understaffed.

When the house supervisor (a mini-Mach) was notified that I needed help, they sat at the desk across from the patient's room and watched as one law enforcement officer and I struggled to subdue the patient. The house supervisor, who was a decades-long experienced RN, made no effort to assist other than to say that someone else would be in to help when they finished their tasks in another unit. No 'code strong' was called, security officers were not employed there at the time, and no physical assistance was offered by the observing mini-Mach. When the officer and I finally had the patient controlled, the house supervisor voluntarily handed me an employee injury report form and said they would "gladly sign it."

Because my injuries were significant and I was unable to work full-duty, I was accepted for the discretionary twenty-six-week state and federal annual Family Medical Leave Allowance (FMLA). Throughout the following six months of recovery and rehab, after having been cleared for light-duty, I checked in weekly with the hospital's employee health nurse and my department manager for any non-bedside nursing jobs.

In addition to my extensive clinical nursing, college instructor, and legal nurse consulting experience the hospital also had an immediate need for a unit secretary, and were looking for additional help to meet the federally mandated 'national digital medical records conversion' (EMR) deadline (both tasks at which I was proficient). I was told there were no "light" jobs available. Even though companies are encouraged by the state's Department of Labor and Industries (workers' compensation) to facilitate an injured employee's return to paid employment, my employer chose not to offer me any alternative options.

Twenty-six weeks later, after a rotator cuff repair and bicep tenodesis (for a dislocated bicep tendon), and treatment for several bulging spinal discs, it was determined that, after eleven years of employment at that particular hospital and a twenty-seven-year RN career, I could no longer work as a bedside nurse. The FMLA law states that if the employer does not provide a light-duty or, in my case, a non-bedside nursing position within the six-month leave allotment, they can terminate the employee.

One day, as I neared the end of my annual medical leave allowance, I received a certified letter. There was no phone call, no acknowledgement of my years of service, no exit interview; just a simple form "termination of employment" letter stating I was "unable to return from FMLA." That was it. My lifelong career of helping, healing, and nurturing others stopped. My life of serving others ended abruptly, and I felt I was no longer needed, or wanted… anywhere.

For reasons still unbeknownst to me the Machs not only wanted me gone, they didn't want me to come back in any qualified capacity. Toward the end of my employment I discovered that much of my personnel file had disappeared. Exonerating documentation, including over a decade of satisfactory to exemplary annual evaluations, reports, and records were gone, and were replaced with a falsified employment history that included substandard performance evaluations I never received.

The word "nurse" is derived from the Latin nutrire which means "to nourish." To nourish someone is the ability "to…supply with what is necessary for life, health, and growth [as well as] to strengthen, buildup, or promote."[55] This is by no means a 'poor me' commentary; it is an illustration of the betrayal I felt by the most trusted profession in the United States: Nursing. Although those who work in the healthcare field are aware of the prevalence of all the 'bad apples', the Gallup Poll (2016) cites that "nurses rank as most honest, ethical profession for the 15th straight year."

I started out decades ago, with a teaching scholarship, as a young university student majoring in

Psychology with a Special Education minor. After spending a summer as a nursing assistant (NA), I decided to change my major to my real passion: Nursing. I have been in the healthcare field since 1971, beginning as an NA and, after a few detours, earned my LPN, and ultimately received my RN in 1986. I have spent the better part of 40 years in service to others and have enjoyed every moment of the journey.

Nursing is what I did, and was a huge part of who I was as I strived to improve and excel in every aspect of my chosen career. Over four decades later, I felt as though my life had essentially ended. All that I am, all that I was, was suddenly taken away from me without any consideration or acknowledgement. Again, a simple "thank you," phone call, or an exit interview would have eased the transition which, without a simple act of common decency, I equated to betrayal. Since that time, I have come to realize that there are people who routinely separate themselves from their inhumane treatment of others, and these morally disengaged people rarely acknowledge their employees even on a good day.

I, like too many other nurses, have not only been the recipient of bullying, but have also witnessed bullying behaviors imposed on colleagues. The bully's unprofessional and inappropriate actions are usually well known not only to the target, but to those who observe their conduct. So, the question that remains is why do bystanders rarely step forward in defense of the victim, making workplace bullying grossly underreported?

Nurse keynote speaker and leadership trainer, Dr. Renee Thompson offers this explanation:

> A study of 1700 health care employees showed that 90% will not speak up in the face of bad practice (behavior), even in life and death situations. If 90% of individuals will not speak up in the face of bullying, bad behavior, and injustice, there must be compelling reasons. [Those reasons include]: Culture of individualism (none of my business, not my responsibility), Fear (how will this person react towards me?), Discomfort (emotion, uncertainty, etc.), Not knowing what to do (caught by surprise, lack of knowledge and practice). ...we are passive and because we are good people, we berate ourselves. Ultimately, because others see our impassivity, the culture of turning a blind eye is reinforced (*When Good People Remain Passive in the Face of Bullying*, March, 2016).

When you add fear of reprisal to the list of reasons nurses do not speak up, silence becomes a job preservation strategy. If there is peer-to-peer bullying, witnesses do not want to become a target themselves. If it is superior-to-subordinate bullying, witnesses risk not only being added to the 'hit list,' they often place their job and entire career in jeopardy by confronting the situation. One reason workplace bullying is underreported is when the victim (eventually) resigns they are commonly blacklisted as unemployable, or "not-for-rehire," to other employers in the region. This is especially true if the targeted employee gives the real reason for leaving in either their letter of resignation or during the exit interview.

The effects of bullying have been well documented and we now know that victims of bullying are at a high risk of suffering long-term psychiatric disorders if the situation is not addressed promptly and properly. Amanda Sounart, associate editor for AMN Healthcare, reports:

> A new study has found that up to 90 percent of nurses have witnessed or were the target of workplace bullying… [and] more than 50 percent of nurses have been the target of some form of abuse at work. According to researchers, nurses who are the target of bullying are prone to developing psychological side effects including post-traumatic stress disorder,

anxiety, depression or insomnia, all of which can lead to poor work performance…many nurses may be unaware of the impact bullying has on them and allow the behavior to continue (*Study Finds Nurses Frequently Being Bullied at* Work, 2008).

Evolutionary anthropologist Hogan Sherrow, Ph.D. (*The Origins of Bullying*, December 15, 2011) explains that "bullying is, in fact, widespread and not restricted to American society, but instead is found across the globe (Smith et al, 2002). From hunter/gatherer groups (Boehm, 2000) to post-industrial Japan, bullying is ubiquitous across human cultures."[56]

Many targets become victims long before they realize they have been put in the bully's crosshairs. All too often, by the time they realize they have been singled-out, targets are already feeling the emotional, psychological, physical, and mental strain of victimization. The transition from being a target to becoming a victim is often quick; it can happen before you know what hit you. The challenge is to recognize that you're being targeted before you become a victim. This can be accomplished by identifying bullying behavior, recognizing who the bully is, and then doing something about it to end the unjust culture before it escalates beyond the point of resolution.

Workplace bullying is becoming better known as experts are looking at all aspects of this type of terrorism. To be clear, "terrorism" includes any organized act of intimidation and fear that is used to coerce the submission of others. In recent years, studies and research of this kind of abuse has accelerated, and the results are published and accessible to all.

From the previous pages in this book, we now have a pretty good idea of the evil that is bullying. And there are steps that can be taken to overcome, or at least deflect, the effects that this terror of repeated intimidation can inflict upon a person.

There are many professional, as well as government, websites available that offer strategic plans to assist those who find themselves targets or victims of bullying. Washington State's Department of Labor and Industries suggests some actions employees can take if they find themselves being bullied:

- Keep a diary detailing the nature of the bullying (e.g., dates, times, places, what was said or done and who was present).
- Obtain copies of harassing/bullying paper trails; hold onto copies of documents that contradict the bully's accusations against you (e.g., time sheets, audit reports, etc.).

- Expect the bully to deny and perhaps misconstrue your accusations.
- Have a witness with you during any meetings with the bully.
- Report the behavior to an appropriate person.[57]

Depending how much time, effort and energy the target (or bystander) wants to invest will determine the effectiveness of documenting the bully's actions, inactions, behaviors, and ethical violations. The quality of documentation (or lack thereof) will either validate the oppressive behavior, or will serve little to no purpose at all.

Following these guidelines, I learned to keep a small notebook in my scrub jacket pocket, and documented pertinent, *objective* information during each shift. I included date, day of week, assigned shift (with start and end time), department staff present, house supervisor name, and so on. Relevant information included start and end times for lunch and rest breaks, how many patients I cared for including their acuity level, and time of admission to time of disposition. The staff with whom I worked knew about the notebook and its purpose. Most of them were aware of the bullying, and many had been targeted themselves.

My quick-reference notebook came in handy many times during meetings with administration and management; especially when I was accused of saying or doing something when I was off-duty. Of all the encounters with my superiors, nothing ever came of the discussions.

It is important to understand all aspects of bullying in order to successfully avoid the long-term effects of this psychologically toxic exposure. Once a target recognizes the signs of bullying, efforts can be quickly focused on remedying, or at least protecting oneself from the hostile work environment; if only I knew then what I know now.

Fueled with a growing and justified paranoia, I progressed to a state of hypervigilance. This was the time I re-grouped and outlined a strategy that included documenting in my black book, and daily transcription of correspondence into my home computer that included e-mails, letters, and telephone messages. Organizing paperwork and documenting in the computer journal was nearly a full-time job in and of itself. At the end of ten months, I had well over a one-hundred-page chronology, including back-up documentation (hard copies), of the inequitable events that were threatening to destroy my career.

What else could be done to stop this insanity? Workplace bullying is not illegal; my union couldn't help because "it isn't in the contract, so there's no violation"; the HR director had done all they could do on their end; and the company refused to honor their anti-harassment policy. There was one last option, so I decided to take it all a step further.

After years of trying to end the unjustified attacks, harassment, and bullying without success, I enlisted outside legal counsel. On advisement, I filed an EEOC protected class complaint citing my manager's comment about me being 'too old to be charge nurse.' Several months later I received a reply that my claims were valid, and I was awarded a Right to Sue (RTS) letter. It had been two long years of consciously battling my superiors, and I was pretty well spent. I was at the point where I wasn't sure if I wanted, or even had the mental stamina, to take on another battle.

It was the words of C. JoyBell C. that gave me the courage to make a smart decision:

> "Choose your battles wisely. After all, life isn't measured by how many times you stood up to fight. It's not winning battles that makes you happy, but it's how many times you turned away and chose to look into a better direction. Life is too short to spend it on warring. Fight only the most, most, most important ones, let the rest go."

I really wanted to let it go and be happy again, so I let it go and began my search for that happiness.

Fighting a battle such as this is not an easy undertaking. When the attacks on me began, there wasn't much information about workplace bullying; or perhaps there was but it wasn't as publicized as it has been in the past couple of years. Blogs and articles, anti-bullying institutes and training, and support groups abound today. And there are innumerable ideas on how to approach the situation if you find yourself a target or a victim. I'd like to say that there's a happy ending to this horrific act of terrorism, but there isn't. There are no laws, punishments, or penalties for those who abuse others through bullying.

As much as I loved my nursing career, circumstances forced me to let it go. Due to a series of events that were never a part of my plan, I have learned that life often goes awry to allow for personal, professional, and spiritual growth.

The truth is that bullying is an act of terrorism and this form of extreme intimidation, regardless of the 'weapon' used, creates a public health and safety threat to both patient and caregiver/employee alike. Until workplace terrorism is recognized as the pandemic it is, efforts to curb its prevalence will be for naught. If left unchecked, I am concerned that what was once thought of as reprehensible behaviors will eventually become globally accepted as the new normal in our places of work, communities, and governments.

For those who are targets or victims of bullying, please know that you are not alone. There are many services available to support and guide you through this crisis. Resources include but are not limited to:

- American Nurses Association's *Incivility, Bullying, and Workplace Violence* position statement (www.nursingworld.org/Bullying-Workplace-Violence)
- *Bully in Sight*: *How to Predict, Resist, Challenge and Combat Workplace Bullying*, Tim Field. 1996
- Bullying Statistics (www.bullyingstatistics.org)
- *Corporate Confidential: 50 Secrets Your Company Doesn't Want You to Know—and What Do About Them*, Cynthia Shapiro. 2005
- NIOSH (www.cdc.gov/niosh/updates/upd-07-28-04.html)
- OSHA (www.abusergoestowork.com/osha-adopts-workplace-anti-bullying-policy)
- RT Connections (www.rtconnections.com)
- Workplace Bullying Institute (www.workplacebullying.org)
- National Suicide Prevention Lifeline 800-273-8255

- Crisis Text Line: text "go" to 741741 (www.crisistextline.org)

If you are being or have been bullied, please remember that "your value does not decrease based on someone's inability to see your worth" (Author Unknown).

Glad Chimp

"There is no reason why good cannot triumph as often as evil. The triumph of anything is a matter of organization. If there are such things as angels, I hope that they are organized along the lines of the Mafia."

~ Kurt Vonnegut

Behaviors devoid of integrity flourish in cultures that tolerate them. Fortunately, there are some ethical leaders, community members, and professional associations that exist to identify, expose, and denounce the growing toxic culture of workplace violence.

Professional organizational efforts to eliminate workplace bullying are on the rise. The American Nurses Association (ANA) is one such agency. The ANA's Workplace Violence Position Statement defines incivility, intimidation and bullying, and describes unacceptable conduct that should not be tolerated. Experts agree that the moment you realize you are being targeted is the time to do something about it; this can include ignoring, confronting or leaving the situation altogether. Research confirms that either confronting the cretin* or resigning your position is the best proactive choice in the long run — for your own self-esteem, confidence, and sanity.

[*Cretin: people whose sole purpose in life is to drain the life-force (i.e. human spirit, positivity, ambition and general well-being) from people whose success in life is related to said character traits.[58]]

Young workers who find themselves on the receiving end of bullying, or are simply miserable in their job, have the option of seeking employment elsewhere, while older or near-retirement age employees have fewer alternatives. Regardless of age, we all have choices, and the ability to change our circumstances. Workplace bullies predominantly target older employees whereby making re-employment challenging at best. As previously discussed, many employers prefer younger and/or inexperienced workers for many reasons; the main incentive being entry-level pay.

I should have divorced my employer long before I had to figuratively die (they were killing me) to escape the abuse. Had I left when I first noticed that something was off, I would never have suffered the devastating effects bullying imposed upon my holistic being. On the other hand, I would not have had the opportunity to navigate through the quagmire of modern-day healthcare, and the ensuing toxic work culture that has befallen tens of thousands of victims and survivors.

Whether the younger or older bullied employee finds another job, or the near-retirement worker retires, rather than wallow in the past it is important to make a conscious effort to hold fast to the present. At the end of his 2016 Olympic swimming career, it was clear that Michael Phelps (at age 31) was at peace with his decision when he announced, "My swimming career might be over but I have the future ahead of me, to turn the page and start whatever I want. It's not the end of a career; it's the beginning of a new journey." This positive perspective holds true at any age. We must move on to the present in order to fulfill our future whether that is with a new employer, or ending one career and beginning a new passion.

My plan was to end this travelogue on an upbeat note — that I achieved victory and all is well. Instead, I must accept the reality that life is often unfair, unforgiving, and unrelenting. To survive this hostile world, gleaning the good in any situation allows us to persevere through the trials and tribulations, and finding the positives in negative circumstances is crucial to attaining victory, or at least maintaining our sanity. This is evident in no better place than our daily work environment.

Survival is a matter of attitude — to find that scrap of good buried under the mounds of negative drivel that is the daily norm. And it is these scraps that enable us to go on and grow on in order to move on from the negative into the positive; if with no other motivation than our basic need to improve the situation, or to remove the situation from our life entirely. There are times when we really do not have any reason to be glad unless we make a conscious effort to embrace the positives in our life.

So, the question remains: how do we achieve that inner peace in a world of contention, condemnation, and emotional chaos? I believe the answer is quite simple yet probably the most spiritually difficult to attain. Knowing we have won, even if we're still in the midst of the 'battle,' is half the challenge.

Regardless of the situation, our mind-set must believe the adversary is defeated; even though this may not yet be the reality. If we fail to declare victory by choosing to live each day downtrodden, then the enemy has won. Victory over our oppressors is a matter of overcoming negative circumstances by focusing on our next success. This requires us to firmly stand our ground with resolve, endurance, and faith, and to remain positive amid the discord and stress. It is our courage, determination, and belief that wins the ultimate battle. Transitioning from victim to victor is not simply a matter of positive thinking, but an act of faith.

This book began as a way to process all that happened to me, and the "65.6 million American employees who are subjected to abusive conduct."[59] The journey started with a look at the early stages of healthcare and, as I traversed through decades of medical advances and hindrances, it ends with the escalation of a centuries-long unjust culture of incivility, intimidation, bullying, and blame. It is my sincere hope that others who are enduring, or have experienced, a similar situation as was mine will feel emboldened and empowered by this book's data and musings.

To paraphrase Maya Angelou, '…I will never forget how the kindness of others made me feel.' It was that kindness from others — family, friends, and strangers — that got me through the toughest times.

As I close this episode of what my life was, I look forward to the next stage of what my life will be.

America's Present and Future State of Health

"It is important to view current events through Christ-like eyes."

~ TODD STOCKER

"AT THE TURN OF THE [20th] century, 2 million chimpanzees lived in the forests of 25 African nations. Today, only 5 nations (Republic Democratic of Congo, Gabon, Central African Republic, Republic of Congo, and potentially Cameroon) have significant populations of wild chimpanzees and their numbers have dwindled to between 150,000 and 300,000 [in large part due to forest encroachment and deforestation]. In the absence of swift action, our closest animal relatives could become extinct..." (Jane Goodall

Institute of Canada, *Conservation & Threats*, n.d.). Just as our primate cousins' very existence is endangered by mostly human interference, mankind's future is equally threatened by their own hand.

This book has presented a few snippets about the history of healthcare, corporate America, and being human. The quest to understand the downward spiral of American healthcare reveals a series of intentional government ultimatums imposed upon its citizens and healthcare entities. Federal demands have generated financial levies that serve to create one of the greatest monetary burdens on the American people, along with stringent industry fines that frequently contribute to an adversarial relationship between the healthcare employer and employee. Adding to this conflict are the interpersonal, agenda-driven divisions which continue to plague the workplace.

The repercussion of America's quasi-national health insurance program has produced devastating effects on its citizenry. Obama's eight year US presidency (2008-2016) produced the advent of the misnomered Affordable Care Act (ACA) under which every American is forced to choose a health insurance plan or face an annual monetary penalty — payable to the US government.

Saving2invest.com (*2016 vs. 2017 Tax Penalty Amounts and Exemptions For Not Having Health*

Insurance Under ObamaCare) presents past, present, and projected federal penalties:

Year	Penalty (Single)*	Penalty (Family)**	Maximum Penalty
2017	$695 or 2.5% of income***	$2,085 or 2.5% of income	$13,100
2016	$695 or 2.5% of income	$2,085 or 2.5% of income	$13,000
2015	$325 or 2% of income	$975 or 2% of income	$12,500
2014	$ 95 or 1% of income	$285 or 1% of income	$ 9,800

* per adult

** $695 per adult; $347.50 per child under 18

*** "dollar amount or percentage of income" denotes whichever amount is higher

Although these fines appear excessive, healthy Americans discovered that the annual penalty is often much more affordable than government imposed insurance premiums.

Obamacare is quickly devolving as several large insurance carriers are opting out of the health-exchange or marketplace program. The remaining insurance companies project a 20% to possibly beyond 116%

premium increase beginning January 2017. Some state exchanges will decrease from several insurers to only one insurance company, and annual deductibles may double — some up to $14,000 per year — while medical coverage is cut in half.

The Kaiser Family Foundation reports that of the 318,868,500 total U.S. population, nearly 156 million (49%) people have "employer-sponsored [group insurance] coverage," 21.8 million (7%) purchase "non-group," or on-their-own premiums, almost 105.7 million are Medicaid (20%)/Medicare (14%) participants, 6.42 million (2%) are described as "other public" who are covered "under the military or Veterans Administration," which leaves nearly 29 million (9%) who are uninsured. (*Health Insurance Coverage of the Total Population*, 2015).[61]

One steep insurance premium increase will be felt by Medicare recipients who subscribe to a Medicare Part D prescription medication insurance plan. Part D plans are offered solely by private insurers who contract with Medicare. Prescription drugs are not covered under basic Medicare Part A (hospital insurance) and Part B (medical insurance).

Beginning January 1, 2017, one particular insurer will increase their Medicare Part D premium by 82 %, some medication costs will increase to as much as 300%, and diagnostic copays will see about a 50% increase. Despite these dramatic increases, Medicare participants were expected to receive the same COLA (Cost-of-Living Adjustment) in 2017 as in 2016 — 0%. It has since been revealed that Medicare recipients will receive a 0.3% COLA. However, in addition to Medicare Part A and B deductible and premium increases (which literally zeroes out the COLA), Part D monthly premiums will, at the very least, double. The paltry 0.3% extra monthly dollars do not begin to offset the exorbitant increase in healthcare costs and monthly medical premiums.

The rising cost of healthcare is in large part because the highest-ranking C-Mach in our nation, President Obama, hedged his bet that Millennials would sign up for Obamacare whereby keeping insurance premiums low for everyone. He counted on healthy young people to defray the healthcare costs of the chronically ill and an aging baby-boomer population. This did not happen. Obama further escalated America's healthcare decline by imposing strict federal regulations, requirements, compliance, and deadlines that include significant financial penalties for non-compliant healthcare corporations.

These edicts, coupled with a host of other financially fueled demands, compound the current convoluted healthcare market. Many health consumers cannot afford insurance under this unaffordable healthcare law. Those who do purchase a marketplace plan can be hard-pressed to cough up doctor visit co-pays, prescription drug costs, and diagnostic radiography or lab fees. Furthermore, deductibles are frequently far too high for the average working, middle-class American.

Although many citizens thought this program might be a bad idea from the beginning, we now know that subscribing to Obamacare, even for basic medical needs, is becoming financially prohibitive. Many healthy Americans are turning to health insurance co-ops and "healthcare sharing" programs instead. These options are less expensive alternatives to conventional health insurance plans.

One healthcare sharing example, which I am not affiliated but am familiar with, is Medi-Share®. Medi-Share started in the early 1990's long before the Affordable Care Act was conceptualized, and it is exempt from current healthcare reform penalty and tax laws. There are many feasible healthcare programs available; however, those who enroll in any insurance plan or program should verify that the carrier is sanctioned under Obamacare's provisions. The plan needs to be federally accepted under the "minimal essential coverage" clause — otherwise, that hefty annual 'non-insured' fine will be enforced. Although there is no immediate solution to the debacle that is Obamacare, there are financially viable alternatives that do meet the federal mandates placed on the American people.

It is mind-boggling that the health of an entire country is sacrificed in the name of democracy, without the foresight to anticipate all possible outcomes — and no Plan B. Many Americans are starting to personally experience that all compassion is lost when healthcare trades beneficence for business...and partisan politics.

The ACA, while it theoretically provides for the expansion of health insurance, also imposes strict reforms on healthcare delivery systems. There are many reimbursement incentives and rewards if regulations and goals are met; however, if these metrics are subpar or deadlines are not met, corporations are penalized with fines, penalties, denial of reimbursement, and other forms of fiscal punishment.

The New England Journal of Medicine (NEJM) points out that "the ACA embraced and accelerated several previous federal efforts to move away from volume-based, fee-for-service reimbursement and to link government payments for health services to providers' performance."[62] Imposing strict regulations and noncompliance penalties on the practice of healthcare (which can jeopardize patient health, care and safety), *Modern Healthcare* magazine found that "the average operating margin in 2013 was 3.1%, down from 3.6% in 2012 based on data available for 179 health systems, which included acute-care, post-acute-care, rehabilitation, and specialty hospital groups and some standalone hospitals. A total of 61.3% of organizations…saw their operating margins deteriorate over the previous year."[63]

Economic demands of the ACA and the Health Information Technology for Economic and Clinical Health (HITECH) Act (which was enacted as part of the American Reinvestment and Recovery Act (ARRA) of 2009) are government regulations that serve to create financial pressure on healthcare entities. The ARRA and HITECH refer to:

> …the national digital medical records mandate for the widespread adoption and use of digital medical records by health care providers. Federal policy initiatives, incentives and reimbursement penalties…are all elements of this national EMR mandate to migrate health care providers to EMR technology. …providers can qualify for Medicare and Medicaid "meaningful use" [incentive] payments [and] can receive as much as $44, 000 [in additional Medicare] payments over a five-year period [and] as much as $63,750 [in Medicaid incentives].[64]

According to the Centers for Medicare and Medicaid Services, "If a participating provider does not successfully...meet "meaningful use" (MU)...he/she will not be eligible to receive an incentive payment for that year...and receiving an incentive payment... is based on the provider's ability to meet MU during that year and not based on success or failure in previous years."[65]

One of the many reforms in the Affordable Care Act (ACA) is another payment incentive that rewards providers who produce "better patient outcomes at a lower cost."[66] One instance of how 'better outcomes' at a lower cost can be attained is when there are no hospital readmissions within 30 days of discharge; otherwise federal penalties will be levied. These "better patient outcomes" are also based on customer service quality rather than quality healthcare; the customers' happiness subverts healthy patient outcomes as evidenced through patient satisfaction surveys, rather than optimum patient *health* outcomes. And the list of government controls and expected goals continue ad infinitum.

As outside financial pressures mount, a healthcare enterprise's primary motivation is to achieve government directives, and increase their bottom line; or at the very least avoid going into the red. Conversely, healthcare workers are focused on evaluating, treating, and helping patients attain and maintain individual health goals. These contrasting objectives can create conflict between the employer and employee, and often trigger contentious conflicts when business subjugates benevolence. Rather than partner with their employees, most employers prefer to rule with an iron fist, or utilize a 'my way or the highway' transactional management style. This practice often leads to adversarial employer-employee relationships, and can contribute to an already volatile work environment.

When we combine the federal demands and fines on the American people and healthcare industries, and add agenda-driven personalities to the work force, interpersonal conflicts continue to threaten the workplace, and patient health and safety. The cumulative effect results in a toxic work environment that is further poisoned by self-serving C-Machs, mini-Machs, and minions; with the triadic goal of promoting themselves by vilifying and eliminating Nightingales.

A wicked and vile web is weaved when no one is available to model morally appropriate behavior and expectations. A transformational leadership style boasts effective leaders who share power, put the needs of others first, and help employees develop and perform as highly as possible. If there is no one daring enough to take a step-out and a step-up to reverse the deterioration of America's healthcare delivery services, workplace culture, and status quo government, then we will soon rue the day when we all had the chance to change the course of history.

The decline of America's healthcare system is but one of the government's many skillfully crafted manipulations intended to generate universal deception; all of which threatens the essence and very existence of humankind. If this cataclysmic course is not corrected, the catapult into pre-apocalyptic Globalization will further demonstrate that not all conspiracies are necessarily theories.

ACKNOWLEDGEMENTS

———

Jesus: my Savior in so many ways.

Saint Richard: my best friend for life and beyond. You are my inspiration. Thank you for always knowing how to make me laugh (especially at myself), and for sticking with me till the day after forever.

Laura: the baby girl of whom I am so proud. Thank you for making a difference in the many lives you touch.

Nathan & Zen: who always beam streams of joy-light into a sometimes dark world.

Zoë Markham: my conscience, editor, and guide who navigated me through this journey.

Acknowledgements

Mr. Armidor "Rocky" Colavecchi: my eighth-grade English teacher whose words I have never forgotten.

ABOUT THE AUTHOR

Having endured six consecutive years in an abusive work environment, PJ found herself in that period of transition from being a victim to becoming a survivor.

For several years, after escaping her tormentors, PJ spent her days as a recovering RN and lived in an alternate reality. It was during this time, when she was not reading, writing, or ruminating, that she found herself longing for the days before nursing and dreaming of someday returning to normalcy.

PJ has made great strides in her recovery. She recently served as an advisor for the American Nurses Association's *Incivility, Bullying, and Workplace Violence* Position Statement, and continues to mentor and inspire nurses. She currently lives pretty much happily-ever-after in the Pacific Northwest.

ENDNOTES

1. http://anthro.palomar.edu/behavior/behave_2.htm

2. http://www.medicinenet.com/script/main/art.asp?articlekey=20909

3. http://www.pasconnect.org/what-is-the-pa-professional-oath/

4. http://www.nursingworld.org/FunctionalMenuCategories/AboutANA/WhereWeComeFrom/FlorenceNightingalePledge.aspx

5. http://en.wikipedia.org/wiki/Nightingale_Pledge

6. http://en.wikipedia.org/wiki/MBA_Oath

7. http://mbaoath.org/about/the-mba-oath

8. *Who's Minding the Store?* Dir. Frank Tashlin. Perfs. Jerry Lewis, Jill St. John, and Ray Walston. Paramount Pictures. 1963.

Endnotes

9. https://essentialhospitals.org/about-americas-essential-hospitals/history-of-public-hospitals-in-the-united-states/

10. http://www.healthmanagementcareers.org/haddock_ch01.pdf

11. http://www.amandagoodall.com/SS&MarticletJuly2011.pdf

12. http://ftp.iza.org/dp5830.pdf

13. http://www.statisticbrain.com/ceo_statistics/

14. *King Kong.* Dir. Peter Jackson. Perfs. Naomi Watts, Jack Black, and Adrien Brody. Universal Pictures, 2005.

15. http://www.remembering4you.com/images/Site-photos/hospital-organizanal-chart.jpg Retrieved June 16, 2013.

16. http://chimpanzeeinformation.blogspot/2009/12/dominance-hierarchy-in-male-chimpanzees.html

17. http://chimpanzeeinformation.blogspot/2009/12/dominance-hierarchy-in-male-chimpanzees.html

18. http://en.wikipedia.org/wiki/Drinking_the_Kool-Aid

19. https://en.wikipedia.org/wiki/Dark_triad

20. http://www.telegraph.co.uk/news/newstopics/howaboutthat/9828914/Why-your-boss-could-easily-be-a-psychopath.html

21. http://www.dailymail.co.uk/news/article-2269154/Horrible-bosses-New-study-shows-modern-offices-reward-narcissism-psychopathic-behavior.html#ixzz2zHHth.XdT

22. http://changingminds.org/explanations/personality/disorders/dark_triad.htm

23. http://www.theglobeandmail.com/report-on-business/careers/leadership-lab/why-are- so-many-managers-useless-as-leaders/article20864299/

24. www.psychologytoday.com/blog/beyond-bullying/201303/surviving-workplace-mobbing-identify-the-stages

25. http://www.vibrantradianthealth.com/author/Cynthia

26. http://www.mayoclinic.org/healthy-lifestyle/stress-management/in-depth/stress-symptoms/art-20050987

27. http://www.healthyworkplacebill.org/

28. *Scary Movie 5*. Dir. Malcolm D. Lee. Perfs. Simon Rex, Ashley Tisdale, and Charlie Sheen. Dimension Films. 2013.

29. http://pin.primate.wisc.edu/factsheets/entry/chimpanzee/behav

30. http://www.forbes.com/sites/hbsworkingknowledge/2013/04/01/first-minutes-of-new-employee-orientation-are-critical/#7b9784251b19

31. http://anthro.palomar.edu/behavior/behave_2.htm

32. https://en.wikipedia.org/wiki/International_Statistical_Classification_of_Diseases_and_Related_Health_Problems

33. https://www.cms.gov/Outreach-and-Education/Medicare-Learning-Network-MLN/MLNProducts/downloads/Hospital_VBPurchasing_Fact_Sheet_ICN907664.pdf

34. www.amnhealthcare.com/latest-healtcare-news/better-nurse%E2%80%93patient-communication-boosts-other-vbp-metrics

35. https://www.studergroup.com/hardwired-results/hardwired-results-03/hardwire-the-five-fundamentals-of-service

36. http://www.ecinsw.com.au/sites/default/files/field/file/Communication%20Talk_AustraliaNSW_EDWorkshop_Smith_Mar2012.pdf

37. http://www.wghblogger.com/2015/05/have-we-been-studerized.html

38. https://en.wikipedia.org/wiki/Customer_service

39. www.merriam-webster.com/dictionary/hospitality

40. www.khn.org/news/medicare-hospital-patient-satisfaction/

41. www.forbes.com/sites/alicegwalton/2012/07/05/bully-pyschology-why-bullying-is-one-of-evolutions-big-snafus/#17280a487f22

42. www.forbes.com/sites/naomishavin/2014/06/25/what-work-place-bullying-looks-like-in-2014-and-how-to-intervene/6a4e97816b41

43. www.who.int/violence_injury_prevention/violence/interpersonal/en/WVguidelinesEN.pdf

44. Dewar, G. 2008. "When bullies get bullied by others: Understanding bully-victims". Parenting Science website. www.parentingscience.com/bully-victims.html

45. Dewar, G. 2008-2013. "Aggressors who are socially-savvy, popular, and smart". Parenting Science website. www.parentingscience.com/pure-bullies.html

46. Sharp, S. 1995. "How much does bullying hurt? The effects of bullying on the personal wellbeing and educational progress of secondary aged students". Educational and Child Psychology, Vol 12(2), 81-88.

47. Aizer, A. ©2008 by Anna Aizer. "Neighborhood Violence and Urban Youth". The National Bureau of Economic Research website. www.nber.org/papers/w13773

48. http://www.livingsafer.com/2013/06/21/when-the-bullied-becomes-the-bully/

49. Parsons, W. 2013. "When the Bullied Becomes the Bully". Living Safer website.

50. www.bullyingsatistics.org/content/adult-bullying.html

51. www.chimpanzoo.org/african_notecards/chapter_10.html

52. http://allnurses.com/men-in-nursing/men-in-nursing-96326htm

53. http://bsntomsn.org/2009/10-most-famous-male-nurses-in-history/

54. www.urbandictionary.com/define.php?term=mean%20girls

55. www.dictionary.com/browse/nourisher

56. http://blogs.scientificamerican.com/guest-blog/the-origins-of-bullying/

57. www.lni.wa.gov/safety/research/files/bullying.pdf

58. http://www.urbandictionary.com/author/php:author=Bob%20Morten

59. www.workplacebullying.org/multi/pdf/WBI-2014-US-Survey.pdf

60. https://www.healthcare.gov/blog/the-fee-for-not-having-health-insurance-2016/

61. http://www.kff.org

62. http://www.nejm.org/doi/full/10.1056/NEJMhpr15036?af=R&ss=curentIssue#t=article

63. http://www.modernhealthcare.com/article/20140621/MAGAZINE/306219968

64. http://www.medicalrecords.com/physicians/the-national-digital-medical-records-mandate-arra

65. https://questions.cms.gov/faq.php?faqid=9220

66. www.commonwealthfund.org/ACAat5/delivery-reform

Made in the USA
Lexington, KY
23 March 2017